T0315437

Praise for Dr. Sharad Paul and his book
The Genetics of Health

"Dr. Paul has been described in the media as 'one of the most inspiring, intelligent, and compassionate men you are likely to meet.' *TIME* magazine, in 2008, called him 'open heart surgeon.'"

New Zealand Medical Association, in awarding Dr. Paul their highest award in 2012

"We need Dr. Sharad P. Paul. In the same sense as the world needs historians-philosophers-sociologists for the history of mankind, the world needs a physician-philosopher-literate for narrative medicine. Only a distinguished physician such as Dr. Paul with a sense for 'stories,' understands the importance of narrative medicine when improving patient-physician communication. He is the Sigmund Freud and Arthur Schnitzler of our times."

Harald Kittler, PhD, professor of dermatology, Medical University of Vienna, and international thought leader in the field of dermatology and skin imaging

"Reading Dr. Paul's book is like taking an exhilarating journey through the shifting landscape of genetics, health, and evolution."

Siddhartha Mukherjee, Pulitzer Prize winner for *The Emperor of Maladies: A Biography of Cancer*

BIOHACKING
YOUR
GENES

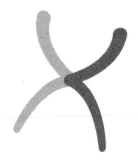

BIOHACKING YOUR GENES

25 Laws for a Smarter, Healthier, and Longer Life

SHARAD P. PAUL, MD

BEYOND WORDS
Portland, Oregon

BEYOND WORDS

1750 S.W. Skyline Blvd., Suite 20
Portland, Oregon 97221-2543
503-531-8700 / 503-531-8773 fax
www.beyondword.com

First Beyond Words hardcover edition December 2024
Sharad Paul IP Limited ebook edition November 2024

BEYOND WORDS PUBLISHING and colophon are registered trademarks of Beyond Words Publishing. Beyond Words is an imprint of Simon & Schuster, LLC.

For more information about special discounts for bulk purchases, please contact Beyond Words Special Sales at 503-531-8700 or specialsales@beyondword.com.

Managing editor: Lindsay S. Easterbrooks-Brown
Editors: Michele Ashiani Cohn, Bailey Potter
Copyeditor: Melissa Ousley
Proofreader: Kristin Thiel
Cover Design: Ryan Butler
Design: Devon Smith
Composition: William H. Brunson Typography Services

Manufactured in the United States of America

10 9 8 7 6 5 4 3 2 1

Library of Congress Control Number: 2024944080

The corporate mission of Beyond Words Publishing, Inc.: *Inspire to Integrity*

For Natasha

Contents

Introduction

Whatever your beliefs—afterlife, reincarnation, or nothing—we are given one life in this human form. Every person on earth has this gift. But without good health, you cannot achieve your true potential.

Today, the online world is so cluttered with health information that even truly scientific health content gets buried under mountains of pseudoscience. The good news is that the internet also allows anyone to reach a wide audience, far away from my medical practice, and that is what this book is about—strategies that are easy to implement and will lead to massive improvement in your health and well-being. All I am doing here is opening your eyes to things I have discovered about the power of your own genes.

The inspiration for this book comes from my patients. Over thirty years, I have seen over 150,000 patients, including famous movie stars, heads of state, and international athletes. But the person who was the inspiration for this book wasn't one of them. Having read my previous book, *The Genetics of Health*, one of my patients, Stefan, wanted to know what I did specifically to look younger, live healthier, and keep fit. He had read in a newspaper article that I had not lost a working day in over thirty years of work as a doctor even though I had worked in hospitals that had treated infectious and tropical diseases. "It's crazy! Doctor, you look at least twenty years younger than your age," he said. Stefan was also astonished to learn that I didn't go to a gym, and most of what I do—diet and exercise— is based on what I have learned over the past twenty years about how we can optimize our genes for better health. Some things were just intuitive, I explained. My lifestyle included a lot of things that my research later found was beneficial. "Just write down things you do," he said. "That's what people want to know."

I have learned many principles from my thirty years as a medical doctor, and these seven are the most important:

1. Medicine is about *illness*, not wellness. Just as law is not justice, medicine is not good health.
2. All healthcare funding is based on medications or procedures for an illness, *not* on prevention.
3. You can take control of your health to make great improvements, and you can start today. It's never too late!
4. We underestimate the power of our genes and how we can *biohack* them for our better health.

5. There is no way you can predict the future, but you can improve your current life. Happiness and health are about *healthspan* not lifespan.
6. You were built to live well. Genes are your blueprint but not your destiny.
7. Whatever habits you have, great health is within your reach, even if it does not seem so at the moment.

With the Human Genome Project came the understanding of the workings of our genes, and understanding our blueprint means we can chart our own health destiny. Charles Weissman, the scientist to first report that genetically modified bacteria produce human interferons—defenders of cells against viruses—said in an interview with *TIME* in 1981, "Biology has become as unthinkable without gene-splicing techniques as sending an explorer into the jungle without a compass."[1]

The major lesson I have learned is that everyone ages. Even "super-agers"—people who live to a hundred and are fit, active, and full of life—still develop diseases that come with aging such as cancers and inflammatory diseases. Except they appear to get these twenty years later than the rest of the population. This book is about how you, too, can become a super-ager.

As a medical doctor who works with skin disorders and cancer every day, I have often been surprised by how people leave major decisions about their health completely to doctors.

When I ask people about their medications, they'll say, "Blood pressure medications," and if I ask them for the names, very few remember the pills they are popping. I often say to them, "So you are putting a chemical into your body, but you don't know what it is?" No one wants less power or control. But when it comes to our health, we seem to push aside our rights and initiative and let others lead us. Where is your health compass? How do you know the health direction you are headed in?

Learning to take charge of your health requires a change of perspective. For example, if one considered our genes to be unmodifiable, then we are trapped inside our biological bodies and there is no reason to try and struggle against them. But genes are just protein makers, and half of the game is in understanding the power of your actions and educating yourself constantly about new insights. Each chapter of this book has specific rules that help us do this better.

I have more than thirty years of experience as a skin MD and physician for celebrities, brands, and major corporations across the world—but most importantly for everyday folk like you and me. I am not an expert in growing a business. But some of those people have everything and yet, nothing. Without health, there is no wealth. Some people call me a health hacker, but I consider myself a lateral thinker, creative, optimist, and—via this book—your personal guide. To follow more of what I do or to get regular health and skin advice, you can follow my blog, *Skin in Your Game*. My blog arose from one of my favorite sayings, which is: "One cannot have bad health and good skin." My mission is simple: to help you biohack your genes for a better life filled with good health, looking your best, and becoming happier by understanding and harnessing the power within your body. This led to the development of the Dermatogenomix® gene-testing program, which is all about how biohacking your genes can lead to better health and wellness.

Go well!

Professor Sharad P. Paul, MD

1

Mind Your Genes

For the energy or active exercise of the mind constitutes life, and God . . . constitutes this energy.

—Aristotle

Chris Hemsworth's Story

Chris Hemsworth is one of the world's highest-paid actors— a super-fit Marvel action hero. Hemsworth actually made *Forbes*'s World's Highest Paid Actors list three times—in 2014, 2015, and 2018. His story began in Australia where he starred in the TV series *Home and Away* before he found fame in Hollywood—starring in films such as *Thor* and *Extraction*.

In the recent *National Geographic* docuseries, *Limitless with Chris Hemsworth*, he explored how we all can unlock our potential to stay fitter, healthier, and happier throughout our lives. Which is really the mission behind this book.

In an episode of *Limitless*, Hemsworth underwent genetic tests to see if he had the risks for any particular disease.[1] As he recalled in the documentary, "his worst fears" were confirmed. He had a higher risk for Alzheimer's disease. Chris Hemsworth's tests revealed that he has two copies of the gene APOE4, one from each of his parents, which means that he has a ten times increased risk of Alzheimer's disease. One in four people carry a single copy of the gene, but less than 4 percent of people have two copies, placing him in the high-risk category for Alzheimer's disease.

In our bodies, apolipoprotein E (APOE genes are the protein makers here) help carry cholesterol and other fats in our bloodstream. We now know that fat metabolism is linked to the development of plaques in the brain that are thought to contribute to the development of Alzheimer's disease. APOE genes come in several forms, what we term as alleles (ε2, ε3, ε4), and each one has a different implication, so is worth understanding:

APOE2

- Percentage of population with this variant: 5–10 percent
- Effect on Alzheimer's disease risk: GOOD

- What it means for your mind: People with this ε2 variant actually develop Alzheimer's disease later in life than normal (i.e., the gene has a protective effect).

APOE3

- Percentage of population with this variant: around 80 percent
- Effect on Alzheimer's disease risk: NEUTRAL
- What it means for your mind: People with this ε3 variant, the most common allele, have neither a decreasing nor an increasing risk of Alzheimer's (i.e., the gene does not make things better or worse).

APOE4

- Percentage of population with this variant: 2–5 percent
- Effect on Alzheimer's disease risk: BAD
- What it means for your mind: People with this ε4 variant have an increased risk for Alzheimer's, and this is associated with an earlier age of developing the disease in certain populations. About 15 to 25 percent of people have this allele, but only 2 to 5 percent—people like Chris Hemsworth—carry two copies.

Alzheimer's disease is the leading cause of dementia in the world. Most cases are sporadic, happening after the age of sixty-five. In medicine, onset after age sixty-five is called late onset! I believe there is plenty of life left if we learn to live well, and those are things that we will discuss in this book. Everyone is worried about losing their minds, and even worse, Alzheimer's disease has no cure at present. We now know that in addition to the genetic profiles discussed here, there are some ethnic differences.

The National Institute on Aging highlighted the importance of ancestry and the APOE4 gene.[2] This was discovered in a landmark study from the University of Miami. The researchers found that if one studied people with both European and African ancestries, it was the genetic ancestry surrounding the APOE gene that determined the risk more than the gene itself. Therefore, if you inherited the APOE4 gene from an African ancestor, you had the African risk for Alzheimer's disease; if you inherited the high-risk variant from a European, you ended up with their risks. So research then focused on differences between ethnic groups.[3] What the studies revealed was interesting and astonishing. For example, the same APOE4 allele in African ancestry populations—irrespective of if they live in Africa or America—carries a lower risk than for European carriers of this gene variant, whereas people with the APOE4 from Asia have a much higher risk for Alzheimer's disease, even more than people of European descent.[4]

The results of Chris Hemsworth's gene test made the Marvel movie star re-evaluate his life and take a complete break from acting for some time. He has been reported as saying: "It's not like I've been handed my resignation.... It really triggered something in me to want to take some time off.... Look, if this is a motivator for people to take better care of themselves and also understand that there are steps you can take—then fantastic."[5]

But as I have always said, science shows that genes are our blueprint but not our destiny. If you have a high-risk variant of the APOE gene, meaning that your chances of developing Alzheimer's disease are higher, there is still hope. More importantly, your actions can determine your destiny. So take charge of your health!

LAW 1

By simply modifying your diet and lifestyle, you can preserve your brain function and avoid developing dementia later on.

The Rhinestone Cowboys

As a lamp is choked by a superabundance of oil, a fire extinguished by excess of fuel, so is the natural health of the body destroyed by intemperate diet.

—Robert Burton

Glen Campbell, the great American singer, songwriter, and guitarist had a string of major hits in the 1960s and 1970s including "Rhinestone Cowboy" and "Wichita Lineman." My dad loved "Rhinestone Cowboy," and we had an old LP he used to play regularly. However, Campbell's first break came when this Arkansas-born musician recorded "Gentle on My Mind" in a studio. The rest is history. But Campbell's lifestyle was not gentle on his mind. In an interview with Larry King in 2002, Campbell discussed his addictions to tobacco, cocaine, and alcohol. Campbell knew intuitively that his body did not metabolise alcohol or drugs well, saying, "I'm a cheap drunk, you know, and I'm a cheap high. I'll put it that way. I could not be around marijuana. I could walk in a room where somebody had been smoking and it would immediately affect me. Because I guess that's the way my metabolism is. Same way with alcohol."[6]

Glen Campbell was diagnosed with Alzheimer's in 2011, the same disease that affected President Ronald Reagan. On hearing the diagnosis, Campbell's family decided to go public and make a candid documentary in 2014, *Glen Campbell: I'll Be Me*, that followed the singer as he dealt with his disease as he went on a farewell tour. His neurologist, Dr. Ronald Petersen, who headed the Mayo Clinic Alzheimer's Disease Research Center, recalled in 2017 about the public display of support from Glen's beloved fans: "The fans came: They loved him. They knew this was going to be the last time they'd see Glen Campbell, and they didn't care if he messed up. If he sang the same song twice or had to stop in the middle of the song—didn't matter. They were there to hear and support Glen Campbell."[7] Glen Campbell passed away on August 8, 2017.

My father, who was once a very respected surgeon, was diagnosed with Alzheimer's disease about seven years ago. He is now a shadow of the man he used to be and is more like a child these days. Such is the fate, in some way or the other, of people when dementia such as Alzheimer's thins away the outer layers of the brain, pokes holes in memory banks, and makes people wonder if this was ever a mind of great eminence. Dad can still hum a mean "Rhinestone Cowboy" tune, though.

There has been very little progress in medications for Alzheimer's disease in the last fifteen years. As Dr. Petersen said, "We don't have to focus totally on pharmaceutical treatments for the disease, because there are certain behavioral and lifestyle factors, things you can do to try to preserve your function as the disease progresses."[8]

The problem is nobody tells you this: I took my dad to an appointment with a geriatrician when he was diagnosed with Alzheimer's disease. Apart from a discussion about Donepezil, an FDA-approved medication for Alzheimer's, there was no discussion about any specific diet. As I researched all the evidence about this medication, I realized that Donepezil does not even alter the progression of the disease, but it can lessen some of the symptoms.

LAW 2

Relying on medications to fix us, without making life-style changes earlier, is like not financially planning for retirement. Taking positive action now saves a lot of heartache (and money) later.

Why Medicines Are Not Always the Answer

A desire to take medicine is, perhaps, the great feature which distinguishes man from other animals.

—William Osler

Over the past two decades, there were regular media reports that a drug for Alzheimer's was just around the corner. The hypothesis most researchers were working on was that the accumulation of amyloid-β was essential to the development of Alzheimer's disease. The theory went like this: extracellular plaques of amyloid, combined with tangles of neurofilaments that extend into nerve cells, caused direct damage and destruction of the nerve junctions (synapses) that mediate memory and cognitive brain function. The building blocks of these structures were amyloid-β peptides for plaques and tau proteins for tangles. Tau was a small biological name for a protein, but it had a big name in research as the cause of many brain diseases including Alzheimer's. In 2014, a paper in the prestigious

Journal of the American Medical Association (JAMA) Neurology even screamed, "Amyloid-β and Tau: The Trigger and Bullet in Alzheimer Disease Pathogenesis."[9] Surely it was a matter of time before a drug based on an enzyme that cleaved the amyloid out of the plaque, or a vaccine-like medication based on antibodies to amyloid-β, would be reality. I had a vested interest in this research because my father's condition was slowly getting worse, so I followed this research closely. But not a single clinical trial worked. Not one even showed a semblance of promise that I would consider for my father. Nada. Not one. Considering that for over a decade all Alzheimer's research had pointed in this direction, it seemed strange that all variations of the theme failed in clinical testing. This pointed to, in my way of thinking, only two possibilities: Could it be that the fundamental hypotheses of so many researchers were wrong? Or worse, was this a case of medical fraud?

Where did this theory about the cause of Alzheimer's disease begin? There was an influential study by Sylvain Lesné and colleagues in the prestigious *Nature* journal that suggested that the amyloid hypothesis of Alzheimer's (i.e., the Aβ clumps known as plaques, referred to previously, in brain tissue) is the primary cause of this devastating illness.[10] This paper, one of the most cited ever in the field, had directed academic and pharmaceutical research funding down this path of searching for drugs to reverse these brain plaques and tangles.

In 2021, an experimental new drug for Alzheimer's disease called Simufilam was about to be launched by a company called Cassava Sciences. But here's where things got murky. A lawyer representing clients who happened to be two prominent neuroscientists—who were also short sellers of stocks, it must be said—believed some research related to Simufilam may have been "fraudulent" and paid Matthew Schrag, a neuroscientist and physician at Vanderbilt University, eighteen thousand dollars to investigate the evidence about this drug.[11] Schrag was deeply concerned to find several altered or duplicated images in dozens of journal articles and alerted the FDA. Cassava Sciences denied any wrongdoing. But this had people wondering—if the drug was based on Lesné's original hypothesis, were the theories about plaques and Alzheimer's disease wrong in the first place? An investigative report in the scientific publication *Science* looked at the evidence and quoted Nobel laureate Thomas C. Südhof of Stanford University as saying: "The immediate, obvious damage is wasted NIH funding and wasted thinking in the field because people are using these results as a starting point for their own experiments."[12]

It wasn't surprising that thousands of people had gone down this research rabbit hole. After all, the first *Nature* paper had originated in the highly regarded research lab of University of Minnesota neuroscientist Karen Ashe—someone who had worked with Nobel laureate Stanley Prusiner on prions, proteins from infections that caused rare brain diseases. Ashe had, in the 1990s, created a genetically modified mouse that produced human amyloid β, which formed plaques in the brain of the mouse similar to human Alzheimer's disease, leading to this hypothesis. She had hired Lesné, a young researcher from France. Lesné discovered oligomers, misfolded proteins in cells, named $A\beta^*56$, abbreviation for "amyloid beta star 56," which—rather miraculously—when injected into mice made them forget information that they knew well, such as locations inside a maze. Ashe's website noted $A\beta^*56$ to be the "the first substance ever identified in brain tissue in Alzheimer's research that has been shown to cause memory impairment." Everything seemed perfect. Perhaps too perfect. In the almost two decades following this discovery, many groups tried to produce this large oligomers $A\beta^*56$, but virtually nobody succeeded to any great degree.[13]

Science magazine asked many researchers to independently review the papers from Ashe's lab. Dennis Selkoe of Harvard University, who had himself copublished with Ashe's group previously but was later unable to replicate findings, examined Schrag's dossier and was quoted as saying, "'There are certainly at least 12 or 15 images where I would agree that there is no other explanation than manipulation.'"[14]

There is no promising drug on the horizon for Alzheimer's disease as I write this book—most certainly, none based on the amyloid plaque hypothesis. This made me disappointed, not as much because of the fraud—as deception occurs in most industries—but because there were millions of people like my father who could have been helped if the past two decades of research had not been wasted.

Current thinking is slightly different with regard to the amyloid hypothesis. Researchers from Ulrich Hengst's lab at Columbia University have found that rather than being the cause of Alzheimer's, beta-amyloid-42 causes two proteins—ATF4 and CREB3L2—to bind together. This pairing of proteins is linked to 50 percent of gene expression changes that happen in brain cells of people with Alzheimer's disease.[15] Therefore, new drugs may emerge that stop the pairing of these two proteins.

There is no point waiting around for a cure that may never arrive. Sure, new medicines for Alzheimer's symptoms will arrive eventually. But for now, you have to take matters into your own hands and heal yourself. We know genes are merely protein makers and our actions—diets and lifestyles—do make a big difference on outcomes. This is even more important in conditions where the science is sketchy or still evolving.

LAW 3

Lifestyle medicine is the new medical specialty where you can be your own doctor.

In this chapter, I am going to talk about the MIND diet and lifestyle changes you can make to reduce your risk of Alzheimer's by more than 50 percent with no medication.[16] That sounds crazy, right? But it is true.

The Power of Movement

Table tennis is like running the 100m while playing chess at the same time.

—Ichiro Ogimura

In science, the best way to realize the power of anything is to understand how life would be without it. As a skin doctor, I have often said that skin reflects our health because it is our oldest and only universal organ. There are animals with no brains (sea squirts), hearts (starfish), or kidneys (Greenlandic sharks), but everything has skin! The importance of movement for brain function is clear when we study sea squirts. These creatures start their life tadpole-like, with a single eye and a tail for swimming. They move around until they find a resting place. Crazily, once these creatures find a home, they literally bury themselves—head down, bum up—and stop moving. But because they become immobile, and a brain is no longer needed for locomotion, these sea squirts literally digest their brains. Adult sea squirts end up brainless, because if one does not need to move or balance, there is no longer a need for an energy-consuming brain.

The brain has three primary functions of movement: grasping, balance, and locomotion. Therefore, we know exercises that include all three of these are best for brain function. While racquet sports and ballroom dancing fit the bill, recent evidence has shown specific benefits of the tango. Why? The Argentinean tango, unlike the waltz or the foxtrot, does not rely on remembered steps. But unlike other dances with partners to grasp on to and that have very little variations in rhythm (I will discuss this closed skill versus open skill later), the tango involves rhythmic variations that participants have to respond to, and therein lies its added benefit. It has been shown to help with dementia as well as symptoms of Parkinson's disease. Studies have shown that the tango could be considered a therapy, as people who danced the tango demonstrated improvements in whole-body positional awareness, improvements in both short-term and working memory, and reduced deterioration of brain function as they aged.[17]

If we said brain stimulation occurs best when we move, grip, and balance, it would follow that racquet sports such as tennis and table tennis should be beneficial. But are they? It turns out they are quite different from the brain's point of view.

Let us look at how our bodies generate energy. There are three energy-producing systems for muscle activity designed to produce ATP (adenosine triphosphate), the energy carrying molecule in all living creatures. We have all heard of aerobic exercise, but interestingly during muscle activity, aerobic systems—because they produce ATP slowly—are triggered only after the phosphagen and anaerobic systems are utilized.

Phosphagen Energy System

Phosphagens are energy-storing compounds that are found in muscles and nerves, which during exercise have rapidly changing energy needs. Therefore, this system has immediate access to reserves of high-energy phosphates that can be used to make ATP. For example, creatine phosphate, which is stored in skeletal muscles, donates a phosphate to ADP to produce ATP.

Anaerobic Energy System

This system is easily explained by thinking about running a one-hundred-meter sprint. Typically, ATP (and thereby energy) comes from glucose through a process called glycolysis, where glucose is broken down into pyruvic acid (pyruvate) through a series of steps. When the body has plenty of oxygen, pyruvic acid is channeled off down the aerobic pathway to be further broken down for more energy. But when oxygen is limited, as in a one-hundred-meter sprint, the body temporarily converts pyruvic acid to lactic acid (lactate), which allows glucose breakdown to occur in order to produce energy. Lactic acid eventually accumulates in muscles and increases the acidity of cells, thereby slowing them down—like easing the throttle—to guard against muscle (engine) damage. Unlike what people think, lactic acid buildup does not cause muscle soreness; however, lactic acid *is* responsible for the burning sensation we feel in active muscles. Once the body slows down, oxygen becomes available and lactate reverts back to pyruvate, and the system changes to an aerobic system. ATP (and thereby energy) in an anaerobic system is produced by converting glucose to lactic acid. This system produces ATP quickly, especially when a surge of explosive power is needed for durations between three seconds to under three minutes.

Aerobic Energy System

The aerobic system—which happens in the cytoplasm and mitochondria of cells—is an oxidative system (i.e., it requires oxygen to produce ATP because carbohydrates and fats can only be fully metabolized to CO_2 in the presence of oxygen). This is primarily used to lower intensity-prolonged exercise after the phosphagen and anaerobic systems have been exhausted.[18]

In table tennis, there is very little lactic acid accumulation. In fact, energy demands rely on the phosphagen system during the fast strokes of rallies (about 2 percent of the total energy expended) and the aerobic system during rest (pause) times (about 96 percent of the total energy expended). Tennis, in contrast, is a predominantly anaerobic activity that also requires a player to have high levels of aerobic conditioning to avoid fatigue. We know from studies that aerobic exercise positively influences episodic memory. EEG studies of table tennis players found greater neural oscillations within the theta band (4–7.5 hertz) in frontal brain areas during table tennis when compared with cycling and other sports, meaning table tennis engages brain regions related to motor control, decision-making, and executive function better than other sports. This brain benefit seen in table tennis is due to it being an open-skill sport as opposed to being a closed-skill sport.

Open skills (i.e., dynamic and changing activities) are typical of table tennis where spin of the ball imparted by different rubber sheets glued onto the paddles (pimpled versus non-pimpled) add variables. I played competitive table tennis once. If someone plays a backspin or a chop, your natural muscle memory in table tennis would either play a backspin back, or preferably, a topspin. However, there are many specially designed "trick" or "funny" rubber sheets that are glued onto the table tennis paddles. For example, Dr. Neubauer Table Tennis is a table tennis rubber brand specializing in such tricky-spin, long-pimpled rubber sheets.[19] However, what happens when you push the ball gently, mimicking a backspin, using these rubbers is this: your opponent sees the racket go down and his or her mind reacts instantaneously—backspin; but your ball goes over the net without spin or even with some topspin! Therefore, more than the serve or stroke technique, there are many other variables in table tennis. It is said that it takes years to overcome the ingrained muscle memory. The world-champion Chinese table tennis teams train to play against tricky paddles by receiving serves through a narrow gap between two curtains so that the receiver cannot see which spin the server is applying; rather, they learn "open skills" by watching the ball move and the bounce.

Closed skills are predictable and static, like those found in archery, golf, running, and tennis, for example. Tennis serves or golf swings are where mastery of the technique or geometry matters, making it more difficult for a beginner to play at a good level. Tennis racquets may be strung to different tension, but they basically are the same materials. In fact, this is corroborated by research studies that have shown tennis players did not have greater executive function and memory performance but instead had better motor skills (i.e., fast reaction times). Gains plateaued when expertise reached a certain level—was better in beginner to intermediate players than at higher levels in tennis, where most people use well-learned techniques such as two-fisted backhands and similar groundstrokes[20]—whereas in table tennis, even expert players have many more unorthodox styles. One only has to watch modern baseline rallies between tennis players. The styles are often similar, and the winner is usually the person who hits the lines the most consistently. This is why during a game of tennis, where baseline rallies are technically similar, mental strength, mindfulness, and the power of analysing an opponent's weakness counts. As Novak Djokovic, the tennis champion, was quoted as saying, "When we are changing ends, when we're sitting on the bench, and then the big screen shows him how he drinks his water. And then I'm looking at him. How is he drinking water? Is he sweating more than usual?"[21]

I have an interest in endurance exercise and the importance of leg movement in the production of brain-derived neurotrophic factor (BDNF). BDNF is essentially a neurotransmitter modulator that helps brain plasticity, making it essential for learning and memory. Open-skilled sports increase BDNF more and reduce the risk of cognitive decline and dementia. BDNF not only makes your endurance better but it also drives brain growth.

If we now consider open and closed skills in the context of dances, we see the tango is open skilled, as one goes with the flow of the partner—who may be a new one every time. In a waltz or the foxtrot, there are well-rehearsed steps, and experts prefer the same partner, as they know the drill. Therefore, ultimately an open-skilled dance like the tango or a sport like table tennis shows the best results for reducing the risk of dementia as one gets older.

LAW 4

Open-skilled exercises that involve leg movement, grasping, and balance such as the tango or table tennis are best for brain function.

Brain Foods

For three million years we were hunter-gatherers, and it was through the evolutionary pressures of that way of life that a brain so adaptable and so creative eventually emerged.

> Today we stand with the brains of hunter-gatherers in our heads, looking out on a modern world made comfortable for some by the fruits of human inventiveness, and made miserable for others by the scandal of deprivation in the midst of plenty.
>
> —Richard E. Leakey and Roger Lewin

The MIND diet was pioneered by Dr. Martha Clare Morris, who was a professor of epidemiology at Rush University in Chicago and director of the Rush Institute for Healthy Aging. Sadly, Dr. Morris died of cancer in 2020. In her early years as a nutritionist and epidemiologist, she noted that people who ate the least amounts of vegetables had the fastest rates of cognitive decline in brain function, but as a person's daily intake of vegetables increased, this decline slowed.[22] If you ate green leafy vegetables six times a week, the effect made your brain eleven years younger![23] Interestingly, eating fruit did not benefit the brain, but berries did.[24] And different berries did different things! When it came to memory, blueberries had the highest positive effect, but when it came to motor function (i.e., movement), strawberries were the best.[25]

LAW 5

Ultimately, it is all about the blood that flows within us. Diets that are beneficial for cardiovascular health have

been also shown to improve cognitive brain function
due to the improved blood flow.

MIND stands for "Mediterranean-DASH Diet Intervention for Neurodegenerative Delay." It is a combination of the Mediterranean and DASH (Dietary Approaches to Stop Hypertension) diets. Let me try and summarize the diet, which along with research from the EAT-Lancet study,[26] gives us plenty of information about brain foods. I like using mnemonics—patterns of letters to help remember a topic—to educate (and remember), so here we go:

A: Avoid These Foods

Avoid red meat and fried or fast foods. If you crave a steak, then try and limit it to once a week. A large cohort study of half a million people showed that each additional portion per week of red meat intake was associated with reduced cognitive function, such as reduced fluid intelligence—involved with processing information or solving problems—and memory performance.[27] Interestingly, in young children and adolescents, it does not make a big difference, but as we get older, red meat worsens brain function.[28]

Also avoid sugars, including artificial sweeteners. In a study from Malaysia, the difference between the twenty-fifth percentile and hundredth percentile of cognitive impairment—memory loss, difficulty in solving problems or concentrating—was three times the sugar intake, with a higher sugar content of 68 to 82 grams of sugar per day (fizzy drinks like Coke contain around 10 grams of sugar per 100 milliliters) leading to the worst outcomes.[29] In trying to quantify this even further, a study from Puerto Rico showed that for every 60 grams of sugar you ate, you dropped 0.4 points in the Mini-Mental-State-Exam (MMSE) used to diagnose Alzheimer's disease.[30] Artificial sweeteners did not fare much better, with research confirming cognitive decline from using aspartame.[31]

B: Berries and Beans

Blueberries are a superfood. In medicine, randomized controlled trials against placebo are the established benchmark of efficacy of a medication, and such a trial was conducted using blueberries by researchers from King's College London and the University of Reading. In a 2023 paper published in the *American Journal of Clinical Nutrition*, sixty-one healthy men and women (ages sixty-five to eighty), drank a drink made from dried wild blueberry powder (equivalent to about 178 grams of whole berries) and were compared against a matching placebo group. The group that consumed blueberries had better memory, greater mental flexibility, and better blood pressure and parameters within twelve weeks! This benefit is attributed to blueberries containing polyphenols, especially strong antioxidants called anthocyanins. Other berries such as strawberries, blackberries, etc., also contain these, but blueberries contain these helpful compounds in the highest quantities.[32] Studies on blueberries have been done on children aged seven to ten with remarkable results. Improved verbal memory, attention span, and reading occurred within two hours of eating the equivalent of 240 grams or one and a half cups of fresh blueberries![33] It is interesting to note that the MIND diet encourages eating berries but does not emphasize consuming fruits in general.

Beans are also very good for you. Eating beans four times a week is recommended in the MIND diet. While all beans, lentils, and soybeans are helpful, there is a caveat when it comes to soybeans: tofu. Studies show high legume consumption seems beneficial in general, but tofu, a soy-based, curd-like product, is associated with detrimental effects by worsening cognitive brain function.[34]

C: Chicken and Poultry

The MIND diet recommends poultry such as chicken (not fried) or turkey twice a week. Studies have shown that eating chicken meat did not have the same worsening effects as red meats did on brain function.[35] In another randomized controlled study, from Southeast Asia and published in *Nutrients*, the benefits of poultry were evaluated by testing the "essence of chicken," a liquid health supplement made from high-temperature and high-pressure extraction of whole chicken. Over two hundred adults were tested after consuming this chicken extract for one to two weeks. The study showed that chicken essence helped the working memory among healthy adults and the short-term memory of adults experiencing stressful events.[36] We have all heard of chicken soup for the soul, but it may also be good for our mind!

D: Dairy

The MIND diet recommends avoiding butter (including fake butter products such as margarine) and cheese. Ideally, substitute olive oil for butter. If you love cheese, try to limit it to one day a week. Here's where the science becomes interesting—as with meat intake, age matters, especially as one reaches "middle life."

I have always spoken about how unnatural it is for the adult of one species to drink milk meant for the babies of another. In fact, milk consumption only began during times of famine and disease. Why do researchers think this? Let's say you are healthy and lactose intolerant. You may get tummy pains and cramps, but you are not going to die from drinking milk. So your genes don't really have to evolve, as there is no pressure. But if your crops and food sources had failed, and you took up drinking milk—due to your poor health, you could die of diarrhoeal disease, so in a proportion of people, genes modify themselves in order to save the species.

Professor Richard Evershed from the University of Bristol studied fragments of pottery and extracted animal fat residues from them to find out where and when people first began drinking milk. It turns out that dairy consumption began seven to ten thousand years ago, which is fairly recent when you consider that our human species has been around one hundred thousand to two hundred thousand years.[37] Genetic studies show that adult lactose tolerance was less common in Roman Britain than today.[38] However, this change was not due to malnutrition but to migration of people from different parts of Europe. Genetic studies of British populations show that people in England and Wales (as opposed to Scotland) have more ancestry derived from these early European farmers. Research has shown that between 1000 and 875 BCE, this European farming ancestry increased in southern Britain (England and Wales) but not in northern Britain (Scotland), where any migrants tended to be people of similar ilk to those from France.[39] Many adults become lactose intolerant as they reach their fifties, and lactose intolerance is also more common in Asians, where ancestral folk were mainly hunter-gatherers.[40] It turns out that even one large glass of milk may be bad for you after middle age. A study showed that having more than one glass of milk a day in people aged between forty-five and sixty-four was associated with a 10 percent decline in global cognitive functioning and memory twenty years later![41] In general, whole-fat foods were worse than low-fat foods. Some studies therefore show dairy in older adults were beneficial, but these were predominantly of the low-fat variety. Consistently, frequency of cheese intake (i.e., the number of times a week you eat cheese) has been associated with decreased cognitive impairment,[42] so having one day a week as your "cheese day" might be a good idea if you are a cheese lover!

LAW 6

Milk may be good for babies but not for adults. Even drinking more than one glass of milk a day during middle age can cause memory loss twenty years later. Limit cheese intake by having a "cheese day" once a week if you wish to consume cheese.

E: Everything Green

The reason green is good is because the green color means lots of heart-protective potassium and vitamin K. Green fruits and veggies also help to maintain vision health and strong bones and teeth. Dark-green leafy vegetables have the highest concentration of antioxidants and fiber.

Green leafy vegetables, such as lettuce, spinach, Swiss chard, and mustard greens, are strongly associated with decreased risk of cardiovascular disease, which, as we know, helps brain function. Cruciferous greens, such as broccoli, brussels sprouts, bok choy, kale, and collard greens, come in a close second. For fruits, the greener ones are more beneficial—green apples are preferable over red. It is interesting to note, however, that some studies have shown that eating fruit appears to have no specific benefit in lowering cancer, unlike vegetables that are linked to a significant reduction in both the incidence and the death rates from cancer.[43] In some studies, fruits and vegetables collectively did not show a cognitive and cardiovascular benefit, but eliminating the fruit—and consuming vegetables alone—had significant benefits. For example, the Chicago Health and Aging Project (CHAP) that was studying Alzheimer's disease looked at a group's combined fruit and vegetable intake for six years and found no benefit, but high vegetable intake showed a significant association with slow cognitive decline, with a further 35 percent reduction in the annual rate of cognitive decline for those top 20 percent vegetable-eaters when compared with the bottom 20 percent.[44]

The importance of green leafy vegetables as brain and mind foods is illustrated by a startling study published in *Neurology* that showed how individuals who have one or two servings of green leafy vegetables every day had a cognitive performance equivalent to being eleven years younger than individuals who rarely or never consumed them![45]

F: Fish

The MIND diet recommends that you eat fish at least once per week. It is best to choose oily fish such as salmon, cod, sardines, trout, tuna, and mackerel that are high in omega-3 fatty acids. Salmon and cod are high in vitamin D also.

As the EAT-Lancet Reference Diet notes, fish contains beneficial nutrients, such as long-chain n-3 polyunsaturated fatty acids (PUFAs), but these days, fish can also be a source of contaminants like mercury and dioxins. We know that mercury can be detectable in hair of those consuming canned fish as opposed to fresh fish, and mercury has been linked to worsening cognition and brain function.[46]

In children, the benefits are clear. Cross-sectional studies have shown that consuming eight grams of fish on average per day in childhood and adolescence improved high academic test scores by one point compared with individuals who consumed little or no fish.[47]

Given the risk of contaminants, studies on fish intake can show variable results. However, a study from the UK on older adults eating plenty of oily fish—not white fish—showed the highest rates of cognitive brain function.[48]

G: Glass of Wine

When it comes to wine drinking, everyone seems to think wine is good for you, but the key is moderation (i.e., not more than a glass a day on average—sorry!). While news reports often claim that wine is good for health, we know that heavy drinking is detrimental for both cardiovascular and brain health. A 2022 study done in Osaka, Japan, used a Japanese version of the Montreal Cognitive Assessment (MoCA-J) and examined older adults after a detailed assessment of their wine-drinking patterns. What they found was a glass of wine one to six days a week was good for you but having non-drinking days was also beneficial. Of the different types of alcohol, wine appears to have some benefit (possibly because of the resveratrol content), provided it is restricted to one glass of wine and not drunk daily.[49] Another study, from

Spain, returned beneficial results associated with moderate wine drinking, but the authors noted that different types of wine need to be studied separately so that consumers could be better educated.[50]

LAW 7

A glass of wine a day has been shown to be good for brain function. However, it is best to limit to one glass per day and have non-wine-drinking days each week.

H: Whole Grains

When it comes to grains, the MIND diet recommends whole grains such as oatmeal, quinoa, brown rice, whole wheat breads (and pasta), and sourdough breads. Whole grains contain resistant starch and are beneficial for the gut and heart, but studies specifically showing the benefits of whole grains for reducing the risk of dementia or improving brain function have been lacking. However, in a Korean study, a positive correlation was found in women older than sixty years, for whom eating whole grain cereals was associated with improved cognitive function that could be measured with the Mini Mental State Examination (MMSE), a screening test used to test for memory loss or dementia.[51]

I: Include These Foods

Try to eat five or more servings of nuts each week. The creators of the MIND diet didn't specify what kind of nuts to consume, but research shows the benefits of walnuts. There was a randomized controlled trial that investigated adults between eighteen years and twenty-five years, and one group was given banana bread with walnuts, and the other, plain banana bread. After eight weeks consuming walnut-containing banana bread, only this group showed a significant improvement in their verbal reasoning skills.[52] Almonds have not shown benefits on cognition, unless they are consumed in quantities over three grams per day.[53] Almonds, among other nuts, are recommended for weight loss because of their low-fat content. A Chinese health and nutrition cohort study showed that individuals who consumed more than ten grams of nuts per day had much better brain function when compared to those who ate less than ten grams of nuts per day.[54] In another study in younger people, a milkshake containing walnut oil improved hippocampal-dependent learning (i.e., retention of knowledge already gained).[55] For example, hippocampal learning involves things like remembering lines in a play or speeches. Even mice studies have shown that walnut intake increased hippocampal function.[56] Human clinical trials have shown an association of walnut consumption with better cognitive performance and memory when compared to baseline in adults.[57]

Another food you should be sure to include in your diet is olive oil. One cannot stress the benefits of olive oil enough. It is preferable to use this as your cooking oil, instead of butter as a spread, and also to drizzle onto salads. Of course, it is often said that olive oil must not be used for frying, but this has not been borne out in studies. It may lose some of its benefits but does not produce harmful compounds as some other oils do. In one study, frying with olive oil increased the trans fat content only by insignificant amounts, and therefore it appears safe even when used as a frying oil.[58]

One of the concerns expressed by researchers is that while there is no doubt olive oil is beneficial, when it comes to reducing the risk of Alzheimer's disease, the concentration of some olive oils may be too low to achieve this. Brain aging is inevitable, so we must do whatever we can do to keep it in top shape. We know that the polyphenols in olive oil reduce oxidative stress in blood cells. Extra-virgin olive oil is derived from the first pressing of the olives, and therefore contains higher amounts of powerful antioxidants and vitamin E, and therefore may be the preferred variety to improve brain function and reduce risk of Alzheimer's disease. Extra-virgin olive oil has shown significant improvement in cognitive functions in research studies, due to its antioxidant and anti-inflammatory action in the brain.[59]

LAW 8

Olive oil is shown to be good for brain and cardiovascular function. Extra-virgin olive oil contains a higher concentration of polyphenols and is the best form of olive oil to use.

Biohacking Your Mind Genes

Given the current lack of effective treatment options for Alzheimer's and dementia, it is important to follow the diets prescribed here if you have a family history of dementia or even for general health. I do not recommend testing specifically for Alzheimer's genes at this time because of the lack of effective treatment options, but this may change in the next few years. Instead, I recommend that everyone follow the MIND diet explained in this chapter.

2

Vitamin D: The Hormone in Hiding

Organized as in us, the hydrogen, the carbon, the nitrogen, the oxygen, those 16–21 elements, the water, the sunlight— all having become us, can begin to understand what they are, and how they came to be.

—George Wald

David Rudisha's Story

In Olympic track events, the 800-hundred-meter dash is considered unique as it lies between a short sprint and an endurance race. In shorter sprints—400 meters and under— you simply go for broke. The 1,500-meter requires you to understand your own pace, the positioning of other runners, and the perfect time to make your move.

In 2012, David Rudisha from Kenya led the entire race to become the first man in history to run the distance under one minute forty-one seconds. Rudisha would go on to win back-to-back Olympic 800-meter races (2012 London and 2016 Rio Olympics) and two world championships (2011 and 2015).[1] His record set over a decade ago still stands. But what makes him so special that I am mentioning him in this book?

As a skin cancer specialist, scientist, and doctor, I know that diagnosing diseases is all about pattern recognition. I have written about how all human skin colors evolved because of the need for folic acid and vitamin D.[2] Simply put, originally skin in Africa was dark to preserve folic acid, and as humans migrated out into Europe, their skin lightened to absorb vitamin D. But the origin of humans in Africa had taken millions of years, and hence evolution had ensured that people in the cradle of human civilization, like David Rudisha, had adequate vitamin D levels.

So, as a bit of a hobby runner myself, I was intrigued with two aspects of David Rudisha's performance and planning, especially the pattern of his time splits when compared with previous legends of the 800-meter such as Steve Cram, Steve Ovett, and Sebastian Coe. When I observed the races of Seb Coe and Steve Ovett, they were typically "kickers" (i.e., these runners typically wait to deploy a devastating and unexpected sprint anywhere between 200 and 100 meters from the finishing line). Because the kick happens suddenly, it is very difficult for other runners to suddenly match this huge increase in tempo. Even though Coe was also a kicker, Ovett's "double kick" essentially made Coe a bystander and—as others have noted—led him to lose the Moscow Olympic 800-meter race to Ovett.[3] Steve Cram, who completed Britain's "holy trinity" of three outstanding 800–1,500-meter runners, had a different training and running style. He was a "winder" (i.e., these athletes essentially wind up the pace around 400 to 300 meters from the finish line with the aim of making the kickers run out of steam).[4] This was the reason why Cram was better in the 1,500-meter, and in fact, he used to train for the 800-meter race on the weekends with a track workout of over 1,500 meters early in the week.

In 2018, Gareth Sandford—who was a PhD student at the Auckland University of Technology where I am an adjunct professor—studied middle distance runners' tactics and their physiological aspects, in association with Athletics New Zealand and High Performance Sport. Sandford's study had some interesting findings about pacing strategies.[5] Firstly, prior to 2015, most athletes employed the "positive pacing" strategy (i.e., ran a faster first lap before the end), and this correlates with the "kick" strategy employed by runners prior to the end designed to outpace other runners into tiring and submission. Secondly, if one was to take the speed of the fastest lap, only one athlete ever in the 800-meter race was approaching nine meters per second: Rudisha—who uniquely was "negatively pacing" (i.e., controlling the race from the start by outsprinting everybody the entire way).

Interestingly, it is believed that Rudisha ran fast from the beginning, which appeared to other runners to be a "positive pacing" strategy. In trying to keep up with Rudisha, six of the seven finalists in the 2012 Olympics ran their personal bests, yet all ran out of steam as this pace was unsustainable to anyone else![6] We know from physiological studies that to accomplish this, someone would need not only a faster speed capability but also unique aerobic and anaerobic energetics. What made David Rudisha different?

There is a one-off documentary called *Man on a Mission* about an Irish missionary, Brother Colm O'Connell, who organized running training camps in Kenya. It was presented by Irish athletics legend Eamonn Coghlan and aired on BBC in 2012. In 2005, a sixteen-year-old David Rudisha ran the 800-meter at one of these camps for the very first time. His time at his first-ever attempt at the distance was only ten seconds shy of his world record ten years later! In fact, in the month he was breaking the world record, he had been supposed to go lion-hunting which was seen as a rite of passage for his Maasai tribe who still lived a traditional lifestyle.[7] These tribes, from whom all of us humans originated, have been shown in studies to have higher average circulating levels of vitamin D. Studies led by Martine Luxwolda from the University Medical Center in Groningen, Holland, have shown that traditionally living Maasai have average circulating blood vitamin D (25(OH)D) levels of 115 nanomol per liter (nmol/L).[8] Until recently, the effect of circulating vitamin D levels on athletic performance was not considered definitive. But now several studies have shown the importance of this miracle vitamin.

However, in 2014, a study was done on Greek professional soccer players to understand the relationship, if any, between vitamin D levels in the blood and muscle strength, aerobic capacity, and speed in these players. What this study showed was that there was a statistically significant correlation between serum vitamin D levels and measured performances in squat jumps, VO2 max (maximum rate of oxygen your body is able to use during exercise), and short-distance sprint speeds. Top soccer players run at top speed intermittently during games, and overall cover ten to twelve kilometers during matches, activities that are directly related to VO2 max.[9] It is clear that circulating vitamin D levels are related to muscle strength, neuromuscular coordination, and explosive movements that are needed for both sprinting and combat sports.

Further, the Maasai tribe consume traditional fermented milk called kule naoto. The *Lactobacillus acidophilus* group strains contained in this showed resistance to gastric juice and bile, meaning this food source is very effective as a probiotic.[10] In 2023, a study of MMA fighters looked at the effect of vitamin D supplementation and directly compared this against vitamin D plus probiotic supplementation. Amazingly, after four weeks of supplementation, researchers found lower lactic acid (lactate) concentrations sixty minutes after acute sprint

runs in the probiotic plus vitamin D group when compared
to the vitamin D group.[11] Lactic acid accumulation causes the
burning sensation in our muscles during intense exercise and
results in slowing down of muscle activity to prevent cellular damage. It appears that Maasai like David Rudisha, living
on a traditional diet full of probiotics and with naturally high
circulating vitamin D levels, are primed for explosive athletic
performance.

In comparison, levels of 50 nmol/L or above of vitamin D
(i.e., less than half of that seen in the Maasai) are considered
good in most people. Recent estimates suggest that 42 percent of Americans are vitamin D deficient (below 30 nmol/L),
with higher levels of deficiency in African American and
Latino populations.[12] In places on the Indian subcontinent,
due to sun avoidance and darker skin, vitamin D deficiency
is even more common, possibly explaining the lack of Olympic track medals. India, with the world's largest population
of one and a half billion people, has never won an Olympic
track gold medal in running (only a field gold medal in jav-
elin throwing)!

David Rudisha stopped competing in 2017 after injuries
sustained in a car crash.[13] His record for the 800-meter set in
2012 still stands. In that race, he completed the 200-meter in
23.5 seconds, the 400-meter in 49.28 seconds, and the 600-
meter in 1:40.91 seconds,[14] and as of the time this book was
published, no other person has ever run the 800-meter under
1:41 seconds.

LAW 9

Athletes with low vitamin D have increased inflammatory markers and reduced performance.

The Autism Anomaly

But unfiltered direct light sort of "needles" its way into the eyeballs of people with autism in sharp straight lines, so we see too many points of light. This actually makes our eyes hurt. This said, we could not get by without light.

—**Naoki Higashida**

I have researched and written about vitamin D for a long time. I have a particular interest in evolutionary biology, especially on how our human skin colors came to be due to the battle in our bodies between folate and vitamin D. But this book is all about how we can biohack our genes and be our best selves and prevent diseases.

I began to think about autism when I had three patients from the Indian subcontinent whose children were diagnosed with autism. I had worked in India for a period but had rarely come across autism. Considering New Zealand's predominantly white population and three cases within a small cohort of Indian subcontinental patients, I began to think about the relationship between autism and vitamin D, especially because studies have shown that Somali mothers who moved to Sweden had greater than four times the risk of having a child with autism when compared to the local homogenous white Swedish population.[15] And, as I have often said in lectures, I have almost never come across Indian patients with high vitamin D levels. Because of vegetarian diets, sun avoidance behavior, and darker skin, there is a high degree of vitamin D deficiency on the Indian subcontinent.

When it comes to autism, research and scientific evidence point to four anomalies and interrelationships:

1. **Rise in autism:** Autism prevalence has risen by 600 percent—indicated by an incidence per 10,000 births of 6.2 in 1990 to 42.5 for 2001 births[16]—in the last fifty years, but this cannot be explained by genetics (i.e., there seems to be no specific gene that is linked to the disease). It is also more common in males, but male hormones do not appear to specifically play a part, but female hormones appear to have a protective effect.[17]

   Furthermore, studies have shown that urbanization increases the incidence of autism. We don't know it this is due to pollution and stress levels that come with city life. The disparities when rural families become urban is more easily studied in countries like China that have large cities that rapidly developed in the past twenty years. Among male children, urbanization has shown a doubling of numbers of autistic children in China.[18] This is not true for female children because estrogen increases brain serotonin synthesis, and this explains why autism is more common in boys.[19]

2. **Serotonin levels and autism:** Brains of people with autism spectrum disorder have significantly less serotonin when compared to people without it. But here is where it gets interesting. Conversely, high levels of serotonin are found in the blood of 25–50 percent of kids with autism. For example, if we took a male child with autism, it is likely that they have high serotonin levels in the blood but low serotonin neurotransmission in the brain. We also know that in individuals with autism, reducing brain serotonin levels leads to worsening of repetitive behaviors and facial recognition issues.[20] I term this the "autism anomaly," or the serotonin anomaly in autism. How can we explain this? Vitamin D.

3. **Vitamin D and serotonin:** The amino acid L-tryptophan is involved in the production of serotonin. L-tryptophan is an essential amino acid. "Essential" in medicinal biochemistry means that it is not made by the body and must be obtained from food (in this instance, foods such as turkey, poultry, eggs, oatmeal, chocolate, etc.; for a detailed list of foods, see the chart later in this chapter). After absorbing

L-tryptophan from food, the body converts some of it to 5-hydroxytryptophan (5-HTP) and then to serotonin. Recently, researchers have identified vitamin D response elements (VDRE) that act on two different tryptophan hydroxylase (TPH) genes that help produce serotonin in functionally opposite ways to one another—inside and outside the brain. For example, one of them induces transcriptional *activation* of tryptophan hydroxylase 2 (TPH2) by vitamin D in the brain, and the other induces reduction of tryptophan hydroxylase 1 (TPH1) in tissues outside the blood-brain barrier by vitamin D.[21] In other words, the action of these vitamin D response elements explains precisely what happens in autism. This vitamin D hypothesis explains why certain states in America have higher autism rates. For example, studies done in the rainy and overcast states of Washington, Oregon, and California on America's West Coast show that children born in places with higher precipitation had higher autism levels, suggesting that more rain means less sunshine and outdoor activity.[22]

4. **Omega-3 and vitamin D on serotonin:** It transpires that when it comes to autism, vitamin D and omega-3 work shows synergies. Most people think omega-3 and fish oils are the same. There are a few subtle points to consider. Fish oil contains two omega-3s

called docosahexaenoic acid (DHA) and eicosapen-taenoic acid (EPA), but natural fish oil contains no more than 30 percent EPA and less than 50 percent DHA, which means the rest is made up of other kinds of fats.[23] Not all fish contain vitamin D. Fish high in vitamin D are oily fish such as salmon, cod, and tuna. Cod liver oil, for example, has around 1,200 interna-tional units (IU) of vitamin D per 15 milliliters, and wild salmon has around 300 IU per ounce.[24]

But the metabolism of fish oil and vitamin D, when it comes to serotonin, has useful linkages, and I believe it is easier to understand them in this way: vitamin D is involved in the *synthesis* of serotonin, EPA helps in the *release* of serotonin, and DHA enhances *uptake* and effectiveness by working on the serotonin receptors in nerve membranes.

Unlike foods consumed by ancient humans, modern diets have too high omega-6 when compared to omega-3. Very high omega-6/omega-3 ratios increase risk of cardiovascular, autoimmune diseases, and even breast cancer.[25] An example of omega-6 fatty acid is linoleic acid (LA), and omega-3 fat, alpha-linolenic acid (ALA). But our bodies cannot manufac-ture these omega-6 LA and omega-3 ALA, and hence these are called "essential" fatty acids that we need from our diets.

Modern cuisines contain a fifth of the omega-3 fatty acids that ancient diets did. For example, our ancestors scavenged the brains of animals that contain DHA.[26] DHA makes up most of the brain's polyunsaturated fatty acid (PUFA) content, and is especially concentrated in the grey matter.[27]

Let's look at essential fatty acids. Our bodies cannot produce one fatty acid in each group—ALA, an omega-3 fatty acid, and LA, an omega-6 fatty acid. These derive their chemical names from the fact that omega-3 fatty acids have a final carbon-carbon double bond in the ω-3 position (i.e., the third bond from the methyl end of the fatty acid), whereas ω-6 fatty acids have it in the ω-6 position. One must remember that ALA is very sensitive to destruction by light, oxygen, and heat, so supplements need to be stored carefully. If not protected, they can turn toxic. ALA is much more easily oxidized when compared to LA.

Both ALA and LA are found in varying degrees in plant and seed oils such as rapeseed oil and walnut oil. In these sources, the LA content is generally higher than the ALA. And arachidonic acid (AA) that is present in egg yolks can be formed from LA. LA is found in safflower, sunflower, and corn oils (high amounts); soybean, sesame, and almonds (medium quantities); and canola, peanut, and olive oils (very small amounts). Palm and coconut oils have generally negligible amounts.[28]

ALA is plentiful in chloroplast and flaxseed oil and present in small quantities in hemp and walnut oils. Flaxseed oil does not convert as easily to EPA and DHA as fish oils do. EPA is abundant in fish oils and both freshwater and saltwater fish. DHA is found in red brown algae as well as fish oil.[29]

What do these fatty acids do? LA is converted to AA, which then forms the phospholipids of cell membranes. ALA serves as substrate in the production of EPA and DHA, which are known for heart and brain benefits respectively.

It is now well-known in medical practice that diets too high in omega-6 and too low in omega-3 fatty acids may lead to chronic inflammation, heart disease, and hypertension, and blood clots.

It's worth noting the benefits of the L-tryptophan–to–competing amino acids (CAA) ratio as it relates to omega-3 fatty acids. The L-tryptophan/CAA ratio indicates how much of the L-tryptophan in the blood is available to cross the blood-brain barrier, where it helps produce serotonin. As I noted, omega-3 fats help reduce inflammation and also improve the blood-brain barrier function. Therefore, lower omega-3 levels affect neurotransmitter function and reduce dopamine and serotonin signaling. Dopamine is our temporary happiness molecule, but it's also involved in movement and coordination. Serotonin is a molecule involved with longer-lasting emotions and mood but also affects gut function and metabolism. So having enough L-tryptophan with respect to CAAs in your diet is crucial for allowing the omega-3s to do their job properly.

L-Tryptophan and Competing Amino Acids (CAAs) Found in Common Foods[30]

	L-tryp-tophan* (mg)	Sum of CAAs** (mg)	Ratio
Turkey, skinless, boneless, light meat, raw (453 g)	410	9,525	0.043
Chicken, skinless, boneless, light meat, raw (453 g)	238	5,122	0.046
Turkey, skinless, boneless, dark meat, raw (453 g)	303	7,036	0.043
Chicken, skinless, boneless, dark meat, raw (453 g)	256	5,492	0.047
Whole milk (946 mL)	732	8,989	0.081
2% milk (946 mL)	551	12,516	0.044
Wheat bread (per slice)	19	317	0.060
White bread (per slice)	22	439	0.050

Semisweet chocolate (28 g)	18	294	0.061
Sweet chocolate (28 g)	16	270	0.059
Tuna, canned (28 g)	472	10,591	0.045
Cheddar cheese (28 g)	91	2,298	0.040
Peanuts (28 g)	65	1,574	0.041
Oats, dried (90 g)	147	2,617	0.056
Prune, dried (one)	2	27	0.074
Banana (one medium)	11	237	0.04
Apple (one medium)	2	70	0.029

The L-tryptophan/CAA ratio represents the relative availability of plasma L-tryptophan for crossing the blood-brain barrier and is thought to be the best indicator of brain serotonin synthesis.

*e.g., The recommended daily allowance for a 79 kilogram (175 pound) adult is 278 to 476 milligrams.

**CAAs = isoleucine, leucine, phenylalanine, tyrosine, and valine, the five large neutral amino acids typically included in the tryptophan/CAA ratio

The role of vitamin D and omega-3 in preventing or managing autism spectrum disorders and mental health cannot be disregarded. Supplementation of vitamin D and omega-3 was studied in a randomized controlled trial of over one hundred children with autism spectrum disorders in New Zealand. After a year, researchers found that *both* omega-3 and vitamin D reduced *irritability* in these children, whereas vitamin D supplementation *alone* was helpful in reducing *hyperactivity.*[31]

Therefore, should pregnant women take supplements to reduce the risk of autism spectrum disorders in their children? A group from the University of California in Davis studied mothers and children after supplementation with omega-3 fish oils. What they found was interesting. The total omega-3 intake of the mother in the second half of pregnancy, especially the second trimester, was statistically associated with 40 percent lower risk of autism spectrum disorder in the child.[32] This may be because the fetus is not able to produce omega-3 fatty acids, which are crucial for brain development, because of their capacity to "occupy 20 percent of the brain's dry weight."[33] Furthermore, omega-3 oils are anti-inflammatory in nature and may reduce neuronal inflammation and thereby irritability. It must be said, however, that in this UC Davis study, the same effect was not statistically seen in the first or third trimesters.[34]

LAW 10

Supplementation with omega-3 oils and vitamin D can help reduce irritability in children with autism and also help prevent the development of autism spectrum disorders if omega-3 oils are supplemented by the mother during pregnancy.

Vitamin D and Skin

If the average man in the street were asked to name the benefits derived from sunshine, he would probably say "light and warmth" and there he would stop.

—Herbert Ellsworth Slaught

The Greek historian Herodotus was not only an amazing chronicler but it appears his observations had astounding medical insights. He wrote about the King of Kings, Cambyses II of Persia (son of Cyrus the Great), who conquered Egypt in 525 BCE in the Battle of Pelusium by defeating the troops of Pharaoh Amasis II. Cambyses requested the pharaoh send him his personal physician and later sought the pharaoh's daughter as a bride. Not wanting to send his daughter to Persia, the pharaoh instead sent over an Egyptian girl named Nitetis, who was the daughter of a previous pharaoh that Cambyses had killed. On learning the truth, Cambyses vowed to destroy Amasis, and this eventually led to the Battle of Pelusium.[35] Later, as Herodotus visited the battlefield, he saw thousands of dead bodies. Herodotus observed that the Persian skulls were so fragile that a pebble was able to break the bone, whereas the defeated Egyptian skulls were so hard that they did not crack even when striking them with a stone.[36] As Herodotus wrote: "The cause of this, they told me, is as follows, and I readily assented; that the Egyptians begin from childhood and shave their heads, and the bone is thickened by exposure to the sun; from the same cause, also, they are less subject to baldness, for one sees fewer persons bald in Egypt."[37]

Herodotus's explanation shows that the ancient Egyptians were aware that something happened that made our bones stronger when bare skin was exposed to the sun's rays. We now know this is vitamin D. Having said this, Herodotus's theory of baldness causing thicker skulls has been commented on in medical circles,[38] but until today, there has been no study that confirms this.

How does our skin produce vitamin D from sunlight? When we expose our skin to sunlight, 7-dehydrocholesterol that is present in skin absorbs UVB radiation and gets converted to pre-vitamin D3, which then becomes vitamin D3 by isomerization.

Over a century ago, Polish biochemist Casimir Funk coined the word *Vitamine* to mean "vita + amine," which later became *vitamin*.[39] Being considered essential and vital for life meant one needed these in our diets. But vitamin D is the odd vitamin out because it is produced by our bodies (via our skin).

Vitamin D is actually a calcium-regulating hormone with endocrine, autocrine, and paracrine functions.[40] The endocrine function of vitamin D is related to calcium metabolism (i.e., controlling serum calcium levels). The paracrine and autocrine functions of vitamin D are involvement in gene transcription, cell differentiation, and cell death, which explains why vitamin D is often low in cancer or deficient immune states. As an excellent article that covers all the different aspects of vitamin D explains, other than bone formation, vitamin D is involved with the proper function of nearly every tissue in our bodies including brain, heart, muscles, immune system, and skin.[41]

In a previous book, *Skin: A Biography*, I differentiated ultraviolet radiation from the sun by their wavelengths in nanometers and what the effects are on our bodies:

- Ultraviolet A: aging (causes wrinkling of skin; implicated in melanoma skin cancers in white skin; penetrates the dermis)
- Ultraviolet B: burning (causes sunburn and tanning in Indian and brown skin types; penetrates epidermis; implicated in nonmelanoma skin cancers)
- Ultraviolet C: cataracts (fortunately, most UVC is filtered out by the atmosphere, but looking directly at the sun is harmful; these wavelengths are especially harmful to the eyes in the Antarctic spring)[42]

As I tell my students, there are myths about sun protection factors. An SPF of 30 in your sunscreen filters out only 4 percent more UV when compared to an SPF of 15 (i.e., 97 percent versus 93 percent). The higher you increase the SPF, the smaller the increase; an SPF of 50 only filters out 98 percent of UV rays. Essentially, higher SPF levels do not mean they have an incrementally higher UV filtering effect. An easy way to remember this is that an SPF 15 sunscreen lets in one in fifteen harmful sunrays, while an SPF 30 sunscreen lets in one in thirty damaging rays, and SPF 50 lets in one in fifty (i.e., offers a 98 percent protection).

At what wavelength is vitamin D produced? Vitamin D production by skin is maximal at UV radiation especially at 295 nanometers (nm). Research shows that if the whole human body is exposed to UVB radiation for fifteen to twenty minutes, your skin is able to induce the production of up to 250 mg of vitamin D (10,000 IU).[43] Of course, in real life, our percentage of body exposure to the sun is far less. In general, I advise my patients to follow the 20:20 rule—20 percent of body surface area exposed to the sun (for example, wearing a T-shirt and shorts) for twenty minutes a day generally gives you enough exposure for optimal vitamin D production. Of course, in places like Australia and New Zealand, where the sun is very harsh with very high UV indices, one needs to be careful of a sunburn, and hence sunscreens are important. One of the concerns with using sunscreens has been the reduction of vitamin D production. But we know that the amount of sunscreen people use is actually too low to block vitamin D production. In my own research lab that makes mineral sunscreens, we also have trialed compounds that aid vitamin D production at a cellular level.

LAW 11

Twenty percent of body surface area exposed to the sun for twenty minutes a day gives you enough exposure for optimal vitamin D production.

How much vitamin D does skin produce from sun exposure? Here are some insights:

Potential Yield of Vitamin D3 Formed in Skin from a Single Exposure to UV Sunlight[44]

	5% skin[a] exposed (mcg)	10% skin[a] exposed (mcg)	20% skin[a] exposed (mcg)
7-DHC[b] at 0.5 µg/cm²	458	917	1834

(continued on following page)

Vitamin D3 produced at 10% conversion	46	92	183
Vitamin D3 produced at 20% conversion	92	183	367

The yield of vitamin D3 in skin, in response to exposure to UV light from the sun, depends not only on the number of minutes of a single period of exposure but also on many other variables, including the seasonal intensity of solar UVB radiation, the absorption of UVB radiation by skin pigmentation, the age of the irradiated individual, and the proportion of pre-vitamin D3 produced that is then converted by prolonged irradiation to other non-biologically active products. Experiments with human skin, irradiated in vitro, have found up to 35 percent of total 7-DHC that can be converted to pre-vitamin D3 in a single exposure session.

[a]Based on the calculated total skin area of an adult male of 18,229 centimeters squared (cm^2).

[b]Lowest concentration of 7-DHC in skin, which ranges 0.5–1.3 micrograms (mcg)/cm^2.

It must be said that vitamin D production depends on number of minutes of exposure but also the intensity of the UV (as too intense UVA radiation actually degrades it), the pigmentation or the skin type, and the age of the individual. Lab studies on human skin models have shown that up to 35 percent of total 7-DHC can be converted to pre-vitamin D3 in a single session of sun exposure.[45]

Humans can only obtain vitamin D from sunlight, diets, or supplements. From skin via sunlight, one cannot overdose on vitamin D as one can if one takes too many pills. This is because all hormones have a feedback loop, and vitamin D is no exception. After less than one minimal erythema dose (MED)—the amount of sun or UV exposure needed to cause pinkness of your skin a day later—pre-vitamin D3 reaches maximum levels. If any further sun exposure is attempted, vitamin D3 gets converted to inactive products such as lumisterol and tachysterol.

The precursor of vitamin D, 7-dehydrocholesterol is found in the plasma membranes of skin cells in the epidermis (keratinocytes) and dermis (fibroblasts). Upon sun exposure, vitamin D3 is produced from 7-dehydrocholesterol and is released from the plasma membrane and into blood circulation bound to a vitamin D-binding protein. Vitamin D levels peak twenty-four to forty-eight hours following exposure to UV radiation and then trail away over the next twenty-four to thirty-six hours. Because vitamin D is considered a fat-soluble vitamin, it is stored in fat cells including inside the abdomen's omentum—the fatty folds of the gut's lining membranes. Once vitamin D enters the circulation after skin production, the liver converts it into 25-hydroxyvitamin D (25(OH)D, or calcidiol), and this is what we measure in the blood to determine vitamin D levels. In general, a level under 50 nmol/L is considered to indicate a vitamin D (25(OH)D) insufficiency. As needed—and controlled by the parathyroid hormone—25(OH)D is converted in the kidneys to an active form called 1,25-dihydroxyvitamin D (1,25(OH)2D, or calcitriol). If one has inadequate 25(OH)D circulating in the blood, or has kidney disorders or other inflammatory conditions, circulating levels of calcitriol are affected.

But in the gut, unlike in skin, vitamin D absorption happens differently. Being fat-soluble, vitamin D gets absorbed along with other fat in the intestines. Chylomicrons, which are lipoproteins that transport fatty acids and cholesterol, also carry vitamin D. And because of the structural similarities between vitamin D and cholesterol, some of the 25(OH)D derived from orally taken vitamin D can become incorporated into VLDL cholesterol that carries triglycerides to tissues. Unlike with skin-produced vitamin D, one can take too many supplements or vitamin D foods and overdose on vitamin D. The main issue becomes hypercalcemia—overproduction of calcium—that can lead to confusion, coma, kidney disease, and muscle weakness and can sometimes even affect the heart.

Unlike from the skin, where only vitamin D3 is produced, one can obtain vitamin D2 (ergocalciferol) or vitamin D3 (cholecalciferol) from our diets or supplements. Vitamin supplements can contain vitamin D2 or D3. So which is better?

Foods such as salmon and cod have vitamin D3. Some mushrooms have vitamin D2, with oyster mushrooms producing twice the D2 when compared with shiitake mushrooms.

Also, mushrooms grown under artificial UV light tend to have higher levels of vitamin D. This is because all mushrooms have provitamin D4 (22,23-dihydroergosterol) and produce vitamin D when exposed to sunlight as humans do, making them a potential source of higher levels of vitamin D if exposed to targeted UV radiation. In general, the D4 levels in mushrooms correlate with the production of vitamin D2, and studies comparing button, oyster, and shiitake mushrooms revealed all had the potential of high levels of vitamin D, even if oyster mushrooms produced the highest levels. A study done in Germany showed that vitamin D2 content of sliced mushrooms was as high as 17.5 mcg/100 g of fresh weight (FW) after fifteen minutes of sun exposure, and it almost doubled to 32.5 mcg/100 g FW after sixty minutes of sun exposure,[46] indicating that mushrooms can tan safer than humans can (see, scientists can make dad jokes too!).

The following chart shows the vitamin D content of unfortified foods. Supplements may contain either D2 or D3. I always recommend D3 because we know from reviews of scientific literature that compared to ergocalciferol (D2), cholecalciferol is better at improving vitamin D serum levels (total levels of 25(OH)D and 25(OH)D3) and regulating parathormone levels, irrespective of the type of person, method (tablet or injection), or dosage.[47]

Vitamin D Content of Unfortified Food[48]

	Vitamin D3		25(OH)D3		Vitamin D2		25(OH)D2	
Reference No.	(6)	(7)	(6)	(7)	(6)	(7)	(6)	(7)
Milk[a] (mcg/L)	0.4	0.08	0.12	0.04	.012	–	–	–
Egg (mcg/egg)	0.55	.072	.03	.024	–	–	–	–
Beef (mcg/100 g)	0.12	0.06	0.17	0.16	0.17	0.027	0.06	0.063
Salmon (mcg/100 g)	8.7	8.7	0.18	0.18	–	–	–	–

[a]Full-cream milk

Interestingly, even with fortified foods and diets containing vitamin D, the seasonal change in populations suggests that sunlight is still the main source. However, many studies that looked at seasonal variations in vitamin D have found that the degree of fluctuation is not significant, even if low vitamin D levels are a global problem with modern lifestyles. A study conducted in Australia on self-reporting adults showed that most Australians could not accurately identify the amount of sun exposure time needed to receive adequate vitamin D levels in both summer and winter, indicating a lack of public knowledge about the amount of time needed to maintain vitamin D levels.[49] However, another study, in Switzerland on young athletes, found that more than half had inadequate vitamin D levels, and this was worse during sun-deprived months. This study also found that taking vitamin D supplements reduced this vitamin D inadequacy during the seasons when there was less sunshine.[50]

LAW 12

Sunshine is still the best source of vitamin D. Of foods, salmon and cod are good sources. In general, sunscreen use does not affect vitamin D absorption.

Vitamin D as an Indicator of Health

Vitamin D may represent the single most cost-effective medical intervention we have today.

—Dr. Greg Plotnikoff

Dr. Greg Plotnikoff from the Penny George Institute for Health and Healing, Abbott Northwestern Hospital, in Minneapolis, has long been a critic of the lack of interest in clinical trials on the benefits of vitamin D. He said, "Let's get a cholesterol test or a blood pressure level . . . That's fine. But it's 20 or 30 years down the road. Vitamin D is something you can replenish and have a return on investment in a couple of months."[51]

I first became interested in calcium metabolism and the importance of vitamin D as a regulator of our health, and indeed skin color in the history of our human species, as I discussed in my TEDx talk, "The Myth of Race."[52] As I discussed in my previous book, *The Genetics of Health*, I find it fascinating that marine invertebrates have vitamin D receptors. Why would sea creatures need vitamin D receptors? Well, because of how it relates to calcium concentrations and how life evolved from oceans to land.[53]

Any creature with a body that contains bone, cartilage, or a shell needs calcium. In general, both animals and plants need calcium. In plants, calcium helps maintain the structure of cell walls and membranes but also is an important messenger between cells. Mitochondria contain approximately 1 nm of calcium, whereas most cells contain around 100 nm (100 billionth of a meter). Seawater contains 400 mg/L of calcium, whereas freshwater's calcium levels are much lower at approximately 15 mg/L. Waters around rocks end up with higher concentrations of calcium, at around 30–100 mg/L, because calcium in rocks can leach out into the water, and this extra mineral raises hardness and pH of the water.[54]

It is not just calcium that is needed structurally but also another mineral, phosphorus, is equally important for bones, teeth, and cellular signaling. However, there is virtually no phosphorus in freshwater or seawater, and it makes phosphorus an "essential" mineral (i.e., needed in our diets).[55] There is a strong and positive correlation between dietary protein and phosphorus (P) in our diets, with organic P found in plant seeds, dairy, fish, and fowl. Inorganic P is found in food additives in processed foods. In certain medical conditions such as chronic kidney disease, high dietary P may worsen hyperparathyroidism, promote calcification of blood vessels, and increase mortality so one needs to be aware of this.[56]

It is no accident that fish that move between freshwater to seawater and back in their life forms, like salmon, have the highest vitamin D levels. Studies have shown that freshwater parr (the fingerling stage of salmon) smolts—or adapts—to seawater, and in seawater adults, plasma concentrations of 25(OH)D3 and 24,25(OH)2D3 did not change significantly. However, plasma calcitriol—the active form of vitamin D—which was lowest in fresh parr, doubled during smoltification (adapting to seawater) and remained elevated in adult salmon in seawater.[57] These dynamic changes indicate that the vitamin D regulatory system plays a crucial role in calcium and phosphorus metabolism in salmon. We know that calcium and phosphorus are important for an optimal immune function, and as the regulator of these nutrients, vitamin D has an important role. In the following sections, I look at the current evidence for the role of vitamin D supplements in heart disease, melanoma, immune diseases, and cancer.

Vitamin D Supplements and Cardiovascular Health

Because I have been talking about vitamin D as a calcium regulator for years, a patient recently asked me if vitamin D affected the "calcium score" of the heart. Let's look at the calcium score, usually called an Agatston score. We know that plaques that clog up our coronary arteries and cause heart attacks are made up of many substances, especially fats, cholesterol, and calcium. Therefore, cardiologists sometimes use a CT scanner to look at the calcium plaque deposits in your arteries. Results are typically reported and interpreted like this:

- 0: No calcium seen in your heart, indicating a very low risk of a heart attack.
- 100–300: Moderate plaque deposits, indicating a relatively high risk of a heart attack in the next three to five years.
- >300: Severe plaque deposits that indicate a very high to severe heart disease and heart attack risk.

Cardiologists also generally report the calcium score as a percentile, which means they compare your calcium levels to other people who are of similar age and gender.

In the past, some observational studies have shown that people with heart disease have lower vitamin D levels. I wrote about the rising incidence of heart disease in the Indian subcontinent and low vitamin D levels in the past.[58] If your vitamin D level is low, calcium leeches out of your bones to try and maintain your cellular calcium, but without a regulator, the task becomes impossible. Vitamin D deficiency leads to calcium deficiency, and when we have low calcium levels, our bodies increase levels of two hormones, parathormone and calcitriol, which increase absorption of calcium from the intestines. This leads to more calcium inside our cells (intracellular calcium). High intracellular calcium levels lead to higher blood pressure and increased cellular fat. This finding—that low dietary calcium raises intracellular calcium—has been called the "calcium paradox," and it has been suggested that it may also play a part in the development of arterial disease and diabetes.[59] However, while this indicates vitamin D is a general indicator of good health, can vitamin D supplements reduce cardiovascular disease specifically?

Recently, a group of researchers looked at twenty-one previous randomized clinical trials in over eighty thousand people. This meta-analysis was published in *JAMA Cardiology* and concluded that vitamin D supplementation was not associated with reduced risks of major adverse cardiovascular events, myocardial infarction, stroke, cardiovascular disease mortality, or all-cause mortality compared with placebo.[60]

Therefore, when it comes to heart attacks, arterial disease, and strokes, taking vitamin D supplements appears to make no difference.

Vitamin D Supplements and Melanoma Skin Cancer

When I have dealt with melanoma—the deadly skin cancer that kills an American every hour[61]—I have noted that patients with advanced melanoma often have low vitamin D levels. This is well-known to people in the medical field, and the assumption had been that the cancer affected the body's "steady state" that vitamin D was maintaining.

However more recently, researchers have considered the following:

1. We know that skin cells are able to activate vitamin D via different pathways.
2. We know melanoma is mostly a cancer of pigmented skin cells.
3. It has been known that in the lab, vitamin D derivatives have anticancer properties.
4. If the above are true, should vitamin D supplements not reduce melanoma incidence?[62]

In 2022, I was invited to speak at the European Academy of Dermatology and Venereology (EADV) Congress, and I saw that one of the posters displayed suggested that people with vitamin D deficiency had poorer outcomes from melanoma than when people had normal levels. For example, if the five-year overall survival rate was 90 percent for a particular stage of melanoma when vitamin D serum levels were above a 10 ng/mL threshold, it dropped to 84 percent when vitamin D levels fell below it.

Very recently, researchers from the University of Finland studied 498 patients who were divided into three groups—low, medium, and high—based on their skin cancer risk by considering skin color, medical history, and other factors. They were also divided into three other groups based on their use of oral vitamin D supplements. The study was well-designed because it had a good representation of the population: ages 21–79 years, 253 males and 245 females, and 96 people with immunosuppression, which we know increases skin cancer risk. Even after factoring in inherent skin cancer risk, the study had some surprising conclusions: People who regularly consumed vitamin D supplements had cut their risk of melanoma by more than half! Interestingly, confirming what we know, that melanin affects melanoma cell susceptibility to vitamin D3 anti-cancer activity—hence the difference in incidence of melanoma between skin types—researchers did not find that consuming vitamin D reduced basal or squamous cell skin cancer rates. However, for melanoma skin cancers, even consuming small amounts of vitamin D appears to be beneficial.[63]

While they could not prove causation, the study confirmed that regular use of vitamin D in a population is associated with fewer melanoma cases and therefore should be recommended as a public health measure in susceptible populations. However, as I mentioned earlier, too much of vitamin D can be harmful, and it is best to not exceed 1000 IU (25 mcg) per day as a supplement. In cases where there is a known deficiency-related disease, then your doctor may recommend twice this amount.

Vitamin D Supplements and the Immune System

In this chapter, I have been focusing on the skin and bone effects of vitamin D. Increasingly, science points to vitamin D as an immunomodulator. We know vitamin D deficiency is associated with immune diseases such as rheumatoid arthritis, systemic lupus erythematosus, and type 1 diabetes.

Vitamin D is involved with the innate immune system, our evolutionary defence system, by its action on skin cells (keratinocytes) and blood cells (monocytes, macrophages, etc.). This was why, historically, from around the 1850s, cod liver oil was used to treat diseases such as tuberculosis and leprosy.

We know vitamin D helps the adaptive immune system also. T cells are cells from the bone marrow that help fight infections and kill cancer cells. In lab studies, we see a specific immunosuppressive subpopulation of T cells, called Tregs, that make the immune system self-tolerant, therefore preventing autoimmune diseases. For example, in research studies looking at inflammatory bowel diseases such as Crohn's and ulcerative colitis, it was noted that vitamin D can enhance Treg function by increasing immunomodulating proteins such as interleukins (IL-10) and CTLA-4, along with tumor suppressors such as TGF-β, thereby suppressing inflammation.[64] These authors also found that vitamin D helped the performance of biological drugs such as infliximab and adalimumab that are used in the treatment of inflammatory bowel disease.[65]

We know vitamin D helps these cells and therefore is useful in potentially preventing and treating autoimmune diseases, especially rheumatoid arthritis. Let's look at some of the evidence here: A large primary prevention trial from Harvard University, published in the *British Medical Journal (BMJ)* in 2022, studied over twenty-five thousand patients with just under a fifth with preexisting autoimmune diseases such as rheumatoid arthritis, polymyalgia rheumatica, autoimmune thyroid disease, psoriasis, lupus erythematosus, etc. This study investigated the supplementation of vitamin D in comparison against vitamin D plus omega-3 fish oil versus a placebo.[66] Vitamin D supplementation for five years, with or without omega-3 fatty acids, reduced the incidence of autoimmune disease by 22 percent (i.e., had a preventative effect). In contrast, supplementation with omega-3 fatty acids alone (without any added vitamin D) did not significantly lower the statistical incidence of autoimmune disease.[67] We also know that vitamin D reduced rheumatoid arthritis activity, and the Comorbidities in Rheumatoid Arthritis study (COMORA) of 1,413 patients in fifteen countries showed that vitamin D levels were inversely associated with disease activity (i.e., the higher the serum vitamin D levels, the better the symptoms or disease scores). There have been other observational studies that have shown that vitamin D either from oral supplements or sunlight exposure could possibly be protective against rheumatoid arthritis. When vitamin D supplementation was tried for osteoarthritis of the knee—our usual wear-and-tear variety—vitamin D supplements only had a modest effect on improving pain and function in patients and did not reverse the disease process, further confirming the specific benefits of vitamin D supplements in autoimmune diseases.[68]

Twenty-four weeks of vitamin D3 supplements also reduced Crohn's disease activity scores in another study— albeit in a small cohort of eighteen patients.[69] While vitamin D levels have been shown to be low in patients with autoimmune diseases such as systemic lupus erythematosus and Sjogren's disease, supplementation has not—to this date—shown any benefit in clinical trials.[70]

Because vitamin D plays a crucial role in immune function and inflammation, during the COVID-19 pandemic, attention turned to the vitamin D status of populations and supplementation. In the UK, there was concern in the NHS about the proportionally large number of infections in non-white medical staff, and a study was undertaken to assess if vitamin D status was involved. The study[71] found that among people with darker skin and a vitamin D deficiency, there was a remarkably high (94 percent rate) of seroconversion—the point from exposure to an infection to when antibodies of the virus become present in the blood due to development of the disease. Another meta-analysis of COVID-19 trials found that while vitamin D supplements were not conclusively shown to reduce the rate of COVID-19 infections, vitamin

D supplements reduced the rates of intensive care unit (ICU) admissions, hospitalization, and death from the disease.[72] Therefore, vitamin D supplements do not stop you from developing COVID-19 but may prevent you from getting terribly ill and ending up in intensive care.

LAW 13

Vitamin D supplementation did not show benefits in cardiovascular disease. However, taking vitamin D supplements may help reduce melanoma and rheumatoid arthritis risk.

Biohacking Your Vitamin D Genes

We know that vitamin D metabolism is encoded by specific genes: CYP2R1 and GC. Vitamin D 25-hydroxylase is the key enzyme that activates vitamin D from its preformed type, which is obtained through sun exposure and the diet. This enzyme is encoded by the CYP2R1 gene and a variant of this gene has been associated with an increased risk of low-circulating levels of vitamin D. The GC gene encodes the vitamin D–binding protein, which binds vitamin D and transports it to tissues. A variant in this gene has also been associated with an increased risk of low-circulating levels of vitamin D.

A study of 180 patients in a family practice in Virginia showed that CYP2R1 (rs10741657) and GC (rs2282679)[73] demonstrated a significant association with vitamin D status. People with one or more variant alleles at rs10741657 were more than three times more likely to be low in vitamin D and subjects with one or more variant alleles at rs2282679 were about half as likely to be insufficient in vitamin D. Allelic variations in CYP2R1 (rs10741657) and GC (rs2282679) affect vitamin D levels but variant alleles on other rs ID numbers—VDR (rs2228570) and DHCR7 (rs12785878)—were not correlated with vitamin D deficiency.[74]

If you have higher risk variants, it is all the more important that you supplement vitamin D daily or increase your dietary intake. To find out your own gene type, your individual risk, and recommendations, you can order your test at www.biohackingyourgenes.com.

3

Folate: For Lasting Health

I was born with spina bifida and should've died in 1951. And they did an experimental surgery in Riley Children's Hospital on me. And they did it to four kids, and I was the only one that lived. And I've never had any trouble with it. But my grandmother . . . said every day, "Buddy, don't forget. You're the handsomest, luckiest, talented boy in the world."

—John Mellencamp

John Mellencamp's Story

John Mellencamp, the rock star from Indiana—who in the past has performed as Johnny Cougar and John Cougar Mellencamp—is well-known for a string of hit songs such as "Pink Houses," "Crumblin' Down," and "Authority Song." In 2014, he released the album *Plain Spoken* that contained the song "Troubled Man."[1] People who hear Mellencamp singing or read about his political activism and Farm Aid concerts—to help families not lose their lands—may not have realized that he was somewhat of a medical miracle child. Mellencamp was born on October 7, 1951, in Seymour, Indiana, with spina bifida[2]—a condition where the neural tube doesn't close all the way (i.e., the backbones that protect the spinal cord don't enclose the spinal cord as they normally should), which can lead to severe nerve damage. While Mellencamp did not have the most severe form of the disease, prior to 1960, the survival rate for all forms of spina bifida—including his type—was only 10 to 12 percent.[3] This was partly because surgeons were reluctant to operate on babies until they were two years old, a conservative medical practice that was later abandoned and eventually led to a marked improvement in early surgery, lesser disability, and reduced death rates. Mellencamp probably would not have survived to become a rock hall-of-famer but for Dr. Robert Heimburger, a neurosurgeon at the Riley Hospital for Children in Indianapolis, who operated on him in 1951. Dr. Heimburger's procedure, considered highly risky in those days, took eighteen hours. Of the four patients that were operated upon, Mellencamp recalled that only he survived into adulthood. In fact, the operation was such a success that John Mellencamp never even knew about the procedure until he finally met the surgeon—when the doctor was ninety-seven—in 2014, more than sixty years later! Mellencamp recalled a childhood friend noting a scar on his back and Mellencamp asking his parents, only to be told, "Oh, don't worry about it.

You had an operation."[4] He assumed he had had a minor procedure, not one that was considered a medical marvel in those days. The surgeon still remembered John Mellencamp because this was the first such procedure he had ever attempted.

During the period when Mellencamp was diagnosed, the importance of folate (folic acid) as a preventer of neural tube defects was not known. These days, almost every person who is pregnant or considering conception knows that an adequate amount of folate in blood helps prevent neural tube defects such as spina bifida in the developing baby.

Marmite, Mumbai, and "Lucy Madam"

Marmite, also marmite
Adjective; British Informal
Causing a strong feeling of either liking or disliking.
Usage: "I think I'm like Marmite; you either love me or you hate me." ~ Lily Allen

—Macmillan Dictionary

A few years ago, after the Christchurch earthquake in New Zealand, manufacture of Marmite (which is very popular Down Under) was halted due to earthquake damage discovered at Sanitarium's Christchurch plant—the only plant where Marmite is made in New Zealand. *The New Zealand Herald* newspaper[5] announced that "Marmageddon" had arrived, and there was a buying and feeding frenzy. The highest bid was for a 1.2 kg jar that was selling for sixty dollars. Ambitious sellers demanded over three thousand dollars for their supply of Marmite. As this was topical as a major news story, I remember telling a patient that while I personally didn't fancy Marmite, it had played a part in a major medical discovery.

In the 1920s, in India (under British rule), Margaret Balfour, who was working at the Haffkine Institute in Mumbai (then called Bombay) had noticed that many pregnant women had developed a severe and often fatal form of anemia. She wondered if this was some kind of a tropical disease. Balfour wrote to the London School of Medicine for Women— England's first medical school for women—because it had an history of academic involvement with India, and her request for assistance attracted the attention of Lucy Wills.

Lucy Wills was a high-achieving feminist who had studied at the elite Cheltenham College for Young Ladies and then at Newnham College at Cambridge—studying botany and geology—before embarking on a medical career. In those days, hematology was in its infancy and was essentially part of clinical or chemical pathology, which my own mother studied after her medical degree. The crisis was initially noted among female textile mill workers. They were dying from anemia, but the cause remained unknown. Wills traveled to India and because most of these women also had diarrhea, initially agreed this was a tropical illness, such as typhoid. The Widal test was already available as a method to check for antibodies against salmonella bacteria that caused typhoid fever,[6] and

Wills wrote: "I spent many hours plating stools and doing Widal tests in an attempt to determine the nature of the diarrhoea and the cause of the high temperature that affected so many of my patients with nutritional macrocytic anemia, only to find negative Widals and non-pathogenic organisms in the majority of patients."[7]

Unable to find a bacterial organism, Wills hypothesized that it was some kind of nutritional deficiency that was causing the anemia. In partnership with some local doctors—Sakuntala Talpade, Robert McCarrison, and Manek Mehta—she decided to try various substances such as liver extracts (considering iron deficiency as a cause) and vitamins A and C (in animal studies on rats) but was unable to come up with an answer. Wills decided to try vitamin B extracts and turned to Marmite. Marmite in those days was made by the Marmite Food Company, which was only too willing to donate some samples for this study. Wills had undertaken earlier lab tests that showed this salty yeast extract was high in vitamins B1 (thiamine) and B2 (riboflavin). Marmite worked in all twenty-two patients that were studied in the trial, curing them of their megaloblastic anemia—wherein anemia occurs because the bone marrow produces stem cells that make abnormally large and therefore nonviable red blood cells. Lucy Wills left India having found a cure, although she was not aware that Marmite also contained vitamin B9 (folate), which was in fact the magic ingredient. She, however, did suspect that there was some other factor when she wrote: "These findings provide further evidence in support of the opinion, expressed in the previous paper, that the extrinsic factor . . . is not vitamin B2 but some other factor, as yet undetermined, which is present in both animal protein and marmite."[8]

The nutritional factor identified by Lucy Wills—at that time named the "Wills Factor"—was later shown to be folate, the naturally occurring form of folic acid that was identified in spinach leaves. Ironically, the link between folate and megaloblastic anemia was published four months after the death of Lucy Wills in 1964.

Folate, which helps the bone marrow produce red blood cells, is usually deficient due to inadequate diets, or sometimes due to issues with absorption caused by alcoholism, inflammatory bowel disease, certain medications, or inherited tendencies. It causes tiredness, pallor, palpitations, and difficulty breathing. Folate deficiency also causes elevated homocysteine levels, which can cause cardiac conditions or cancer.

LAW 13

Folate supplementation reduces neural tube birth defects and megaloblastic anemia and is now standard medical advice during pregnancy and preconception.

Homocysteine and the Heart

> He had been invited to a conference of heart specialists
> in North America. . . . Next morning Best looked round
> the breakfast room and saw these same specialists—all in
> the 40–60-year-old, coronary age group—happily tucking
> into eggs, bacon, buttered toast and coffee with cream.
>   —Richard MacKarness

Sheryl Sandberg, the inspirational tech executive and former
Facebook chief operating officer, wrote *Option B: Facing Adversity, Building Resilience, and Finding Joy* along with Wharton
professor Adam Grant—a book to help people dealing with
adversity after the loss of a loved one develop resilience. In the
part-memoir, part-self-help book, Sandberg talked about the
loss of the love of her life, Dave Goldberg, and how she learned
to find meaning after this personal tragedy.[9]

Dave Goldberg, Sandberg's husband, was only forty-seven
when he passed away unexpectedly while on a family vacation
in Mexico. He had been exercising on a treadmill and fell. As
Sandberg later confirmed, the cause was not the fall but undiagnosed coronary artery disease that had led to an arrythmia
of the heart.[10]

As a doctor with a keen interest in preventative healthcare
and wellness, I was interested in this story because I had been
researching folic acid, its impact on homocysteine levels and
increased health risks caused by low folate—especially heart

attacks in middle-aged individuals. Folate deficiency causes high homocysteine levels that make middle-aged men more prone to heart attacks. Of course, I do not know the details of Goldberg's medical history. But recently a study was done of middle-aged men in Taiwan to look specifically if any association between homocysteine levels and cardiovascular disease risk existed.[11] What the results revealed was that elevated homocysteine levels are an independent risk factor for heart disease in middle-aged to elderly men. Higher homocysteine levels were associated with higher cardiovascular risk with a odds ratio (OR) of 2.499. An odds ratio of greater than 2.0 indicates a more than double risk of these men developing heart disease.

More recently, in May 2023, Indian TV actor Nitesh Pandey died of a sudden heart attack. He was fifty-three. In an article in the *Indian Express* newspaper reporting of his death, Dr. Venkat Nagarajan, a cardiologist from the Kokilaben Dhirubhai Ambani Hospital in Mumbai, was quoted as saying: "As per the Indian Heart Association, 50 per cent of all heart attacks in Indian men occur under or at 50 years of age. Most of the deaths are from sudden cardiac arrest (SCA), a condition where the heart stops working without any warning. This occurs when the electrical signals that coordinate the heart's beats don't work appropriately and may be the first presentation of a heart attack."[12]

What made the heart attack risk higher in India? Was it purely to do with bad diets and sedentary lifestyles when compared with Mediterranean countries, for example? Was this something metabolic? Did homocysteine levels have anything to do with this? A major medical laboratory chain in India, Tata 1mg Labs, undertook a population survey spanning the whole of India. What this study revealed was both suggestive and alarming. As was reported in the *Times of India*, "More than 66% of people in India have higher than normal levels of homocysteine in their bloodstream, making them vulnerable to heart diseases, such as blood clots, heart attack and stroke."[13]

This wasn't only on the Indian subcontinent. Almost two decades ago, researchers in Japan had also sought to investigate their relatively high stroke rates among middle-aged people and had concluded that total homocysteine concentrations in the blood were associated with the increased risk of strokes, more specifically ischemic strokes, among both Japanese men and women.[14]

Mendelian randomization studies are types of analyses where researchers look at genetic profiles and how people with a particular genetic profile may react to a particular environment, drug, or behavior. These clinical studies are often done to overcome the biases that can occur in an observational study. For example, "information bias" may result from incorrect recording of individual factors, such as risk factors or the disease being studied. The other kind of bias could be a "selection bias," where people chosen for a study could already have a particular ingrained behavior such as being more health conscious or physically active. In a Mendelian randomization study, because the genetic profile is already known, it follows that any genetic differences are not influenced by selection bias and reflect a true prolonged or lifelong difference. Such studies are increasingly popular in cardiovascular research.

An influential Mendelian randomization study assessed the association of serum homocysteine levels and vitamin B (folate (B9) and B12) levels with cardiovascular diseases in the general population. This study, led by Susanna Larsson of the Unit of Cardiovascular and Nutritional Epidemiology of the Karolinska Institutet in Sweden, showed that genetically predicted higher folate (vitamin B9) levels were addition-ally associated with a lower risk of coronary artery disease, whereas the same association was not noted with vitamin B12 levels. The study also showed that supplementing with folate to reduce homocysteine levels reduced the incidence of stroke and possibly heart disease, as had been noted in other stud-ies. The researchers noted that taking folate as a therapy to lower homocysteine levels may even play a role in the preven-tion of stroke, especially ischemic strokes and possibly ones caused by subarachnoid bleeds.[15] Previously, we had looked at vitamins in Marmite that had helped reduce megaloblastic anemia in pregnant women and birth defects. Folate and B12 are both known to be present in Marmite; we now know that folate reduces risk of vascular disease and vitamin B12 does not.

Another study[16]—this time a meta-analysis—led by Frank Hu of the Harvard T. H. Chan School of Public Health looked at thirty randomized controlled trials involving more than eighty thousand participants that had previously reported on using folate supplements to reduce homocysteine levels in the blood as a means to preventing cardiovascular disease. This meta-analysis indicated that folic acid supplementation caused a 10 percent lower risk of stroke and a 4 percent lower risk of overall cardiovascular disease. However, there were two important observations. Firstly, the effect was more pronounced for those with no preexisting heart disease but where high homocysteine levels had been lowered by the folate supplements. Secondly, in those that already had established coronary artery disease, there was no difference (i.e., folic acid did not help unclog arteries). This means that high homocysteine levels increase the risk of heart disease in previously healthy people and taking more folate can help reduce this risk. But when one looks at strokes, the evidence is more straightforward—the risk of an event was reduced by folate supplementation to reduce homocysteine levels irrespective of disease status.

We know that folate is the biggest dietary factor that influences homocysteine levels in the blood. Research now indicates that taking between 0.4–5.0 mg of folic acid typically lowers plasma homocysteine levels by approximately 25 percent.[17] Therefore, research suggests that folic acid supplementation must be recommended to any patient or person who has an elevated homocysteine level, and this level should be measured and treated at an early age because folic acid is so easily available as a supplement and could end up preventing these people ending up with strokes or heart attacks.

But what is homocysteine, and what is the relationship between folate and this amino acid?

LAW 14

Folate supplementation must be recommended to anyone who has a high homocysteine level, as it may prevent heart attacks or strokes.

The Link Between Folate and Homocysteine

When physiologists revealed the existence and functions of hormones they not only gave increased opportunities for the activities of biochemists but in particular gave a new charter to biochemical thought, and with the discovery of vitamins that charter was extended.

—Frederick Gowland Hopkins

Folate, or vitamin B9, helps in the production of red blood cells (hence the anemia we discussed earlier), DNA synthesis, and methylation reactions. The active form of folate once it is absorbed from our intestines via our food becomes tetrahydrofolate, which is considered the backbone of one-carbon reactions that make folate a major generator of cellular NADPH, a veritable powerhouse. The active form of folate is 5-methyltetrahydrofolate (5-MTHF), which is a methyl donor (remethylation) in the conversion of homocysteine to methionine, another amino acid. Methionine, in turn, contributes to the production of S-adenosylmethionine (SAM). This SAM is involved in methylation reactions (i.e., donates its methyl group to various other molecules, including DNA and neurotransmitters). This link to DNA synthesis is why folate and methionine metabolism are increasingly studied in cancer and longevity research. Methionine is an essential amino acid that we get from protein-rich foods such as fish, meat, beans, and nuts and is involved in the production of glutathione. Glutathione is a major antioxidant found in most cell types, and increasingly, researchers interested in epigenetics are looking more closely at this tripeptide made up of three amino acids (cysteine, glutamic acid, and glycine) that needs sulfur to be produced. Glutathione is both an antioxidant and a detox agent.

The remethylation reaction mentioned earlier—where homocysteine is converted to methionine—is the reason folate and homocysteine levels are linked. The enzyme methionine synthase transfers the methyl group from 5-MTHF to homocysteine, producing methionine, a reaction that also needs vitamin B12 as a cofactor. Folate is effectively a recycling agent for homocysteine by converting it to methionine.

Methionine is an antioxidant that helps rid the body of toxins after ionizing radiation or drug overdoses, for example. But if someone has low folate levels, then this conversion of homocysteine to methionine cannot occur, leading to an accumulation of homocysteine. And as we discussed earlier, having high homocysteine levels means a higher risk of nerve development defects, strokes, and heart disease. But how do high homocysteine levels cause heart disease?

The link between folate-related genes and homocysteine levels has also caused some controversy in medical circles. Methylenetetrahydrofolate reductase gene (MTHFR) variants cause high homocysteine levels and demonstrate the importance of folate supplementation or dietary augmentation for people with high-risk variants.[18] However, one meta-analysis[19] had shown that while folate supplementation did reduce homocysteine levels, it did not reduce the risk of cardiovascular disease, making many doctors unsure of the benefits of folate. Therefore, recent research has focused on trying to understand the mechanism by which high homocysteine levels affect the heart. Laboratory studies have previously shown that elevated homocysteine does increase reactive oxygen species (ROS) (i.e., free radicals) production in microvascular endothelial cells, leading to inflammatory responses within blood vessel walls.[20] Many studies have also shown the clear link between elevated homocysteine in the blood and calcification within blood vessels of the heart and brain.[21] Recently, research published in the *Journal of the American Heart Association* for the first time showed the clear link between high homocysteine levels and worsening of calcium deposits within arterial walls, which we know leads to plaque formation. This multi-ethnic cohort study was interesting because baseline homocysteine measurements and cardiac computed tomography (CT) scans were studied for over six thousand people and followed up with further assessments. The authors concluded: "This is the first study demonstrating an association between elevated homocysteine and both incidence and progression of coronary and extra-coronary vascular calcification. Our findings suggest a potential role for elevated homocysteine as a risk factor for severe vascular calcification progression."[22]

Research in a new study now points to the role of high homocysteine levels as a risk factor for the worsening of blood vessel calcification that we know leads to coronary and vascular disease, and further studies in the future will make this picture clearer.[23] I know what I would personally do; I wouldn't wait around but ensure that with adequate folate, my homocysteine levels are not high.

LAW 15

High homocysteine levels are a risk factor for the worsening of calcification in blood vessels, and therefore, keeping homocysteine levels low is important, and this may involve folate supplementation.

Folate, Cancer, and Longevity

It infiltrates everything. It's metastasis. It gets into every single pore of productive life. I mean there won't be anything that isn't made of plastic before long.

—Norman Mailer

Norman Mailer may have been talking about plastic, but there is a chemical connection between plastic and life forms: carbon bonds. Plastic is a polymer of long carbon chains. For example, plastic bags begin as ethylene, which is treated to become the polymer form, thereby creating long chains of carbon and hydrogen atoms. Carbon is also the basis for all life everywhere on Earth, because it helps form complex molecules like proteins and DNA. Being critical to the foundatons of life forms does not mean a loyalty to a being. If one looks at the domain of biochemistry philosophically, carbon ends up being both precise and prophetic. Today we know that a significant amount of industrialized microplastic and nanoplastic particles are present everywhere in our environment and implicated in a wider variety of cancers in human body systems.[24]

As a skin doctor who deals with skin cancer daily, I've learned two things:

1. Cancer is essentially our immune system at its best and most hyped persona.

2. Most people, even those we may consider are old, want to live longer.

Therefore, cancer research and longevity advances are intricately linked. After all, cancers are also more common as we age, as we are past our reproductive peak and our genetic machinery begins to malfunction.

As our solar system and planets were formed, carbon-based life forms evolved on our planet. Why did carbon (and not silicon, for example) become the chosen element for life? We don't know. But we know that any life form needs energy to function. Every living creature therefore needs an agent and systems to release this energy and utilize this energy created. In our human environment, or indeed for all animal forms, we have oxygen as this agent, and during cellular respiration, glucose—because it functions as a carbon-based energy source—is broken down, producing CO_2 and H_2O, and energy is released. Cells produce glucose without us consuming glucose sugars, from sources such as proteins and fats. The by-products of this carbon life, CO_2 and H_2O, can be easily eliminated or recycled in our metabolic systems. If life had evolved around silicon—it may have elsewhere in the universe—the chemical reactions would have happened at different temperatures. These temperatures would be far higher than what our human forms can survive in, and therefore, we are unlikely to encounter such alien forms. Further, such a life form could not be oxygen dependent as we are because when silicon reacts with oxygen, it forms a stable lattice that is not excretable by the metabolic or chemical systems we are familiar with. The flexibility of carbon or its innate ability to form bonds with other atoms or biological biomolecules such as nucleic acids (RNA and DNA) means that life—as we know it—is impossible without carbon. And that brings us to one-carbon metabolism, which has folate as its basis. Let's imagine one-carbon metabolism as a series of building blocks that are used to maintain essential structures and organs within our bodies. Folate becomes the veritable LEGO®—the most efficient one-carbon donor—ensuring that building blocks are properly assembled and useful when finally built. These one-carbon units are carried to where they are needed within a cell by small molecules such as folate and other coenzymes. Understanding this one-carbon metabolism is so important in both cancer and longevity research, so let's consider this further (and I apologize for this chemistry lesson but will try and simplify things).

Essentially, folate can transfer single carbon atoms in three different oxidation states: methyl (CH_3-), methylene (CH_2-), and formyl (CHO-).

- **Folate as methyl (CH_3-) donor:** Methylation involves donating a methyl group to specific molecules, which can modify their structure and function. DNA methylation is particularly important as it is the mechanism by which genes are turned on or off. The importance of this is self-explanatory given genes are our blueprint.

The single carbon donor 5-MTHF (5-methyltetra-hydrofolate) is used to convert homocysteine into methionine, which can then be used to methylate DNA. We now know that differential methylation as well as disturbances in nucleotide synthesis and repair are associated with several forms of cancer. For example, hypermethylation of tumor suppressors is involved in the progression of benign tumors like adenomas to cancerous forms. Another way of simplifying this is understanding that methylation of a gene switches it off. The more methyl groups added onto a gene, the more securely turned off that gene is.

- **Folate as methylene (CH2-) donor:** In its methylene guise, folate carries a single carbon atom bonded to two hydrogen atoms (CH2-). This form of folate is involved in the synthesis of thymidine, a key component of DNA. We know that thymidine is essential for both DNA production and repair. As a skin doctor, I can explain this in a practical way: Our skin only becomes sunburned when ultraviolet radiation causes thymine dimers to be produced at a rate that overwhelms the repair mechanisms. In addition to tanning our skin in an attempt to protect it, thymidine dinucleotide induces a photoprotective response, by enhancing repair of UV-induced DNA damage.

- **Folate as formyl (CHO-) donor:** In its formyl form, folate carries a single carbon atom attached to one hydrogen and one oxygen atom (CHO-). This form is useful in producing amino acids, especially serine and glycine. Serine is not only involved in protein synthesis but also in the making of cellular signalling molecules. Glycine has anti-inflammatory, antioxidant, and immune-protective actions and helps produce important compounds such as glutathione, porphyrins, purines, haem, and creatine.

Diet and One-Carbon Metabolism

Choline and folate are linked through their involvement in the one-carbon metabolism pathway as methyl donors. Choline is metabolized to betaine, and betaine can donate methyl groups in reactions that require one-carbon units. Folate provides its own methyl groups in the form of 5-methyltetrahydrofolate (5-MTHF). A nutrient that plays numerous roles such as lipid transport and regulating brain and nervous system functions, choline is needed for the production of acetylcholine, which is a neurotransmitter implicated in memory, mood, and muscle control, and other brain functions. Choline is a vital structural component needed to form cellular membranes and impacts early brain development and regulates the function of genes, or how they are expressed.

Methylenetetrahydrofolate dehydrogenase (MTHFD1), a gene that encodes an enzyme responsible for folate (also known as vitamin B9) metabolism, is also implicated in choline metabolism because MTHFD1 (along with another

PEMT) gene also impacts dietary choline requirements. My explanation of this may be found at the end of this chapter.

Caenorhabditis elegans (*C. elegans*), the nonparasitic nematode worm, is one of the best-studied organisms for studies of cell behavior and death and also in human longevity research. This is because it is a one millimeter-long soil worm that can live in petri dishes and contains just over one thousand cells. Even more, its transparent body makes it easy for observing its cells that are remarkably constant in location and numbers, making it also an excellent model for metabolome research.[25]

Metabolome research has advanced significantly now. The metabolome represents the totality of the number of by-products from metabolism such as calcium or water, found in life forms. Because metabolism is essentially everything that happens in a cell, studying the metabolome can give us insights into health status, disease progression, response to environments (diets or lifestyle), and lifespan. In fact, metabolomics is a science that uses scanners to look at these biochemical processes happening in real-time, and the *C. elegans'* transparent body makes this easier. Recently, a paper in the influential *Nature Communications* journal used high-resolution mass spectrometry to identify potential metabolomic pathways that regulate lifespan in *C. elegans*.[26]

When it comes to longevity, researchers found that one-carbon metabolism and the folate cycle is the common regulator of these life-extension pathways. We discussed homocysteine earlier and how methylation of homocyste-ine completes the methionine cycle (even if homocysteine can also be channeled into transsulfuration, glutathione, and pyruvate pathways). It now transpires that a key to living longer is metabolic methionine restriction. Dihydrofolate reductase (DHFR-1) carries out two chemical reaction steps, firstly reducing folic acid to dihydrofolic acid (DHF) and then to the active form of tetrahydrofolate (THF). This enhanced activity is because this polyglutamate form of folate remains trapped in the cell, thereby prolonging its action for longer. When genes that control this enzyme DHFR-1 were studied in the *C. elegans* worm, these genes increased mean lifespan by 28 percent.[27] Even drugs like metformin, the biguanide anti-diabetic drug, are being tried in some life extension clin-ics because they restrict methionine.[28] Methionine restriction therefore appears to have a profound effect on physiology and regulates longevity through multiple mechanisms.

I am a big believer and promoter of healthspan rather than lifespan (i.e., living to your full physical and mental potential to the very end as opposed to merely looking at the number of years lived). For your healthspan, your biological age mat-ters. Biological age tells you where your system is at age-wise as opposed to your chronological age that is based on your birthdate. It is indeed possible to be sixty years old and have a biological age of thirty. But how do we measure this? By using an "epigenetic clock" that is based on the levels of DNA meth-ylation. How is this done? By measuring DNA methylation in several different cells and tissues and at different locations on someone's DNA, and then by using some computerized algorithms, one can determine that person's biological age. Such research already shows that lifestyle matters—because heavy drinking and smoking rapidly increases your biological age, whereas healthy eating reduces this. I mentioned earlier how vitamin B12 is needed as a cofactor in the reaction where the enzyme methionine synthase transfers the methyl group from 5-MTHF to homocysteine, producing methionine. Given methionine restriction in the metabolome increases lifespan, one can expect benefit from supplementation of related B vitamins. This brings up the question: Do vitamin B9 (folate) and B12 (cobalamin) decrease biological age?

One study in 2018 analyzed forty-four adults for two years after supplementing with vitamins folate (400 mcg/day) and B12 (500 mcg/day). The results showed that, after supplementation, women who carried the normal genetic variants for methylation activity had epigenetic clocks that were running slower than those of others (i.e., supplementation had slowed the aging process).[29]

Telomeres: Our Cellular Timekeepers

Also related to the aging process of cells are telomeres—the protein bits that stick out at the ends of our chromosomes—which become shorter each time a cell copies itself, while the important portions of the DNA stay intact. Every time a cell divides by mitosis, the telomeres shorten, and once telomeres shorten to a critical length, the cell can no longer divide. Telomeres are effectively biological clocks within each cell that quietly tick away and have therefore been considered our cellular timekeepers (i.e., biological clocks that measure our real age). It has been suggested that low folate levels could lead to shorter telomeres by removal of increased uracil in the telomere which leads to more DNA breaks.[30] This was the rationale behind studying folate supplementation.

A randomized study of over five thousand people from the National Health and Nutrition Examination Survey (NHANES) looked at the dietary B12 and folate levels across multiple age groups and ethnicities, so that the results would be applicable across the US population. Firstly, telomere lengths were measured using polymerase chain reaction (PCR). Then dietary folate and vitamin B12 were measured using twenty-four-hour blood levels. What the study found was interesting. For each additional year of chronological age, telomeres were 15.6 base pairs shorter on average. Men had shorter telomeres than women overall, which explains why women generally live longer than men. Serum and dietary folate concentrations were linearly related to telomere length in women, but not in men, after controlling for age and race. In other words, irrespective of gender or age or ethnicity, folate made a meaningful difference in slowing cellular aging in women, but not in men. Vitamin B12 made a much smaller difference, but again this difference was noted in women only.[31] In attempting to understand this difference between men and women, the main theory is that men have a lower response to folic acid because in general, men have a larger body size and therefore the dose of folic acid distributes over a larger volume. Furthermore, a lean body mass also affects folate levels. In most studies, men indeed had a higher dietary folate than women but needed more folate to achieve the same concentration of folate within red blood cells (which is the most accurate measure of folate status). Therefore, the recommended daily intake of folate should be higher for men than for women.[32] In other words, it may be more important for men to supplement folate than women, but this hypothesis needs testing because, in clinical studies thus far, only in women do folate supplements appear to slow down biological aging.

LAW 16

Folate supplementation in the diet can help slow down biological clocks in females. Both micronutrients folate and vitamin B12 help, but folate seems to be the most important.

Biohacking Your Folate Genes

The MTHFR gene produces methylenetetrahydrofolate reductase, which is a vital enzyme for folate metabolism in the body.

MTHFR converts folate from our food to an active form of the nutrient that can be used by the body at the cellular level. Variations in the MTHFR gene determine the way individuals respond to dietary folate.

We know that some people who have the CT or TT variant of the MTHFR gene have reduced MTHFR enzyme activity and are at greater risk of folate deficiency when folate intake is low, compared to those with the CC variant. For these individuals, it is particularly important to have high folate foods.

Food Sources High in Folate[33]

Sources of High Folate	Folate Content (DFE)
Lentils, boiled, salted (146 g)	265
Edamame (82 g)	255
Spaghetti, cooked (148 g)	184
Spinach, boiled, drained (95 g)	139
Asparagus, boiled, drained (90 g)	128
Chickpeas (garbanzo beans), canned, not drained (175 mL)	119

Black beans, canned, not drained (175 mL)	108
Broccoli, boiled, drained (82 g)	89
Avocado (101 g)	81

Note:

1 DFE = 0.6 mcg folic acid from dietary supplements consumed with foods

1 mcg DFE = 0.5 mcg folic acid when supplements are taken on an empty stomach

And in general, I would recommend a folate supplement of 400 mcg daily for those looking at optimizing their biological clocks. The evidence is greater for women at present, but the jury is still out as more studies are being done.

MTHFD1, the methylenetetrahydrofolate dehydrogenase gene, also encodes an enzyme responsible for folate (also known as vitamin B9) metabolism. Choline's function seems to be linked to the metabolism of folate, as they share overlapping roles in the same metabolic pathways. People who carry the A allele of this MTHFD1 gene are at higher risk of developing clinical signs of choline deficiency—muscle damage, liver damage, and non-alcoholic fatty liver disease—when choline intakes are very low in comparison to those who have the GG genotype.

The PEMT (phosphatidylethanolamine N-methyltransferase) gene encodes a protein that allows the liver to produce choline. Individuals with the CG or CC variants of the PEMT gene are at a higher risk of experiencing clinical signs of choline deficiency compared to those with the GG variant if choline intake is low. For these high-risk individuals, increasing choline in the diet is especially important.

Food Sources High in Choline[34]

Sources of High Choline	Choline Content (mg)
Egg, hard boiled (1 large)	147
Soybeans, roasted, salted (120 mL)	107
Chicken breast, roasted (85 g)	72
Ground beef, 93% lean meat, broiled (85 g)	72
Atlantic cod, cooked, dry heat (85 g)	71
Baked red potato, flesh and skin (1 large)	57
Wheat germ, toasted (28 g)	51

Kidney beans, canned (120 mL)	45

If you have higher risk variants, it is all the more important that you supplement folate daily or increase your dietary intake.

4

OILS: THE GOOD, THE BAD, AND THE UGLY

The first oil of all, produced from the raw olive before it has begun to ripen, is considered preferable to all the others in flavour; in this kind, too, the first droppings of the press are the most esteemed, diminishing gradually in goodness and value.

—Pliny, the Elder

Gary Beauchamp's Story

In the previous century—all right, it was only 1999!—Gary Beauchamp, a noted psychobiologist from the Monell Chemical Senses Center in Philadelphia, was in western Sicily at a molecular gastronomy gathering attended by physicists, chemists, biologists, chefs, food writers, and others interested in the science of sensation. Ugo Palma, the convenor of the meeting, had arranged a tasting session of freshly pressed extra-virgin olive oil from his family's farm. As Beauchamp recalled: "I sniffed and savoured and swallowed as directed by Ugo. While the oil was in my mouth, it gave a soft and not entirely pleasant oily impression. When swallowed, it slid down smoothly. But, a few seconds later, I felt a strong stinging or burning sensation in the back of my throat. This burning sensation grew in strength until I coughed; others in the group coughed in concert."[1]

This extra-virgin olive oil tasting got Beauchamp thinking. In the 1990s along with his colleagues, he had been working with a drug company developing a cold and flu remedy, Lemsip. Lemsip is widely available in the UK and Commonwealth countries like New Zealand and is essentially paracetamol (or acetaminophen) along with a decongestant. But when the company had attempted to replace paracetamol with ibuprofen (or add ibuprofen), people complained of bitter taste, and hence Beauchamp's team that researches the perception of taste was engaged. Paul Breslin and Barry Green from Monell found that ibuprofen caused a different type of throat irritation to capsaicin (found in chili peppers) or carbonation and wondered if anti-inflammatories such as ibuprofen had specific throat receptors. They also found that if the pH of an ibuprofen solution was made more alkaline and raised above seven, the throat burn went away, but the drink was no longer lemony, and so Lemsip, to this day, still contains only paracetamol.[2]

However, this story has an interesting twist. When Beauchamp returned from his trip with a bottle of this extra-virgin olive oil, Breslin asked him why he had added ibuprofen to the oil because the bitterness of the oil had a similar bitterness to the anti-inflammatory medication. Were the two linked (i.e., does a specific medicinal property indicate a special taste)? Other researchers had also begun to look at compounds in olive oil and separate out the bitter-tasting chemicals and had noted that the bitterness of olive oil was due to aglycones, specifically the dialdehydic and aldehydic forms of oleuropein aglycone, and dialdehydic and aldehydic forms of ligstroside aglycone.[3]

When the Monell team ran studies on the compound that made olive oil bitter, they found that it was indeed a natural anti-inflammatory compound with a potency slightly better than that of ibuprofen! Therefore, they concluded that anyone on a traditional Mediterranean diet consuming this extra-virgin olive oil would be taking a daily anti-inflammatory dose from extra-virgin olive oil that could be considered the equivalent of low-dose aspirin. And, true to their discerning taste buds, Gary Beauchamp's team had discovered the anti-inflammatory action of extra-virgin olive oil and the mechanism (i.e., like ibuprofen) of oleocanthal in extra-virgin olive oil dose-dependently inhibits COX1 and COX2 enzymes as many anti-inflammatory and anti-arthritic drugs do.[4]

Olive oil has two groups of compounds: saponifiable (soapy) lipids (98–99 percent of the total composition) and an unsaponifiable fraction. The main saponifiable triglyceride fatty acid is oleic acid, which makes up 55–83 percent of the total fatty acid content.[5] It also includes moderate amounts of palmitic and linoleic acids and a low percentage of stearic and linolenic acids. The unsaponifiable fraction contains a large variety of compounds that include squalene and phenolic compounds that include tyrosol, hydroxytyrosol, and oleocanthal.[6]

I will discuss the cardiovascular aspects of olive oil in more detail in the next section. Tyrosol and hydroxytyrosol are phenolic compounds found in all olive oils; hydroxytyrosol is indeed one of the main phenolic components of olive oil, and it is known to protect and lower low-density lipoproteins and consequently reduce cardiovascular disease risk. However, the bitterness we have been discussing of extra-virgin olive oil is due to oleocanthal, and we know this has several health benefits. While oleocanthal constitutes only around 10 percent of the total phenolic component of extra-virgin olive oil, its impact is far greater.[7] In addition to the anti-inflammatory effect we discussed, oleocanthal is now showing promise in anti-Alzheimer's and anti-cancer research. For example, my work involves skin cancers such as squamous cell cancers. Oleocanthal has shown promise in lab studies against human epidermoid carcinoma cell lines and increasing cancer-cell death.[8] Studies on breast cancer cells in the lab showed a similar benefit where oleocanthal downregulated estrogen receptors in breast cancer cells, thereby suppressing the growth of hormone-dependent breast cancer and working alongside medications such as tamoxifen used for such cancers.[9] Oleocanthal also reduces the protein buildup in Alzheimer's disease and oleocanthal-rich extra-virgin olive oil has been shown to enhance the effectiveness of donepezil (a medication used for Alzheimer's disease) by reducing amyloid-β loads, albeit at present this has only been shown in mouse models.[10]

Basically, extra-virgin olive oil, obtained from the cold pressing or centrifugation of the olives, is the one with highest content of total phenolic compounds. Virgin olive oil has a total phenolic content of 232 mg/kg, whereas refined olive oil has 62 mg/kg because almost 80 percent of phenolic activity is lost in the refining process.[11] As some researchers have noted, while not all benefits are due to oleocanthal, its bioactivity is greater than what the other phenolic compounds in standard olive oil can manage.[12] It appears that extra-virgin olive oil, due to the added oleocanthal compounds that cause its bitterness, has a greater benefit than other olive oils against a multitude of diseases, and I would advise people to use extra-virgin olive oil preferentially over the other varieties.

LAW 17

Out of all varieties of olive oil, extra-virgin olive oil is the most medicinal with anti-inflammatory, anticancer, and anti-dementia properties.

The Good Fats and Cholesterol

It may one day be possible for many people to have their
steak and live to enjoy it too.

       —Michael Brown and Joseph Goldstein

Fats are useful in the diet because they help in the absorption
of the fat-soluble vitamins (vitamins D, E, K, A). Each gram of
fat provides more than twice the calories on a gram per gram
basis. This makes fat an energy-dense food. If we considered
this from an evolutionary biology perspective, our brain—
essentially a super-computer—has high energy demands and
that led humans to consumer denser foods when compared to
primates. Further, we know that key long-chain polyunsaturated fatty acids that are critical to brain development.

    However, we also know that the amount and types of fats
that we eat affect both our heart health and body composition.
As a general rule, unsaturated fats are heart-healthier than
saturated or trans fats. But here we need to consider some
genetic elements. For example, the TCF7L2 gene is involved
in body weight regulation and body composition. We know
from research that people with the TT variant of TCF7L2
experience greater weight loss when they consume lower to
moderate fat diets, as opposed to when they consume higher
fat diets. For those people with the CC or TC variant, there is
no difference in weight loss irrespective of the fat consumed.[13]
We see this often in people who say they lost weight on higher-

fat and lower-carb diets, even if for weight loss one needs a lower total energy intake to create a calorie deficit.

In the previous section, I discussed the benefits of extra-virgin olive oil. What makes olive oil good is that it is a mostly unsaturated fat. When it comes to fat consumption, unsaturated is good; saturated is bad. Now let's look at some finer aspects. When I am speaking at wellness festivals or at events educating the public about good health and eating, I am often asked questions about coconut oil because some people on paleo diets prefer this. Many people consider it a healthy fat. How does it compare with olive oil?

Coconut oil is mostly saturated fat. The easier way to know if a fat is saturated or not is to simply look at the fat at room temperature in its unrefined state without additives. If it solidifies like coconut oil or butter, it is mostly saturated. The predominant type of saturated fat in coconut oil (which is almost 90 percent saturated fat) is lauric acid at almost half, with myristic and palmitic acids in smaller amounts.[14] All these have been shown to raise LDL (bad) cholesterol levels. The counter argument is that plant-saturated oils are not as bad as animal saturated fats, although cardiologists are concerned that coconut oils cause significantly higher LDL cholesterol than nontropical vegetable oils, and advise coconut oil restriction in the diet.[15] In fact, in countries like New Zealand where doctors have restricted access to medications, a few years ago a patient needed a certain LDL level before a doctor could prescribe a statin. I remember meeting a cardiologist who used to get his patients to consume coconut oil to push the levels higher to qualify for a statin before taking the coconut oil out of their diets! He believed that plant-based fats did not clog arteries as these sterols have a chemical structure that mimics blood cholesterol and may actually block the absorption of cholesterol in the body. However, the amount of these sterols found in a few dozen milliliters of coconut oil is too small to produce a beneficial effect overall for health. Therefore, if you want the benefits of coconuts, then eat the fruit, not the oil. Coconut oil does have some medium chain fatty acids that are absorbed quickly after metabolism by the liver, but lauric acid, the main component, is a longer-chain fat and metabolized more slowly. If we look at countries where coconut oil is traditionally used, such as in India and parts of Asia, people eat the whole coconut as coconut pieces or press the pulp into coconut cream, and the diets are high-fiber vegetable diets with very little processed foods. The less processed or refined an oil is, the better it is for health.

Food Sources High in Saturated Fats[16]

Sources of Saturated Fats	Saturated Fats (g)
Ice cream, vanilla, premium (125 mL)	11.7
Short ribs, lean + fat, simmered (75 g)	11.2

Cheddar cheese (50 g)	10
Butter (5 g)	7.5
Regular ground beef, crumbled, pan-fried (75 g)	7
Cheeseburger (1 patty, plain)	6.5
Whole milk (250 mL)	5.4
Muffin, chocolate chip, commercial (1)	5.3
French fries (20–25)	5
Salami, beef and pork (46 g)	3.7

We have to understand that all oils may contain a mix of saturated and unsaturated fats. In olive oil, the majority is unsaturated, mainly monounsaturated. In contrast, other oils considered healthy such as fish oils, flaxseed oils, and sunflower or soybean oils contain omega-3 or omega-6, which are polyunsaturated. Olive oil contains mostly monounsaturated fat—as a rough guide, ten times that of coconut oil; as a ballpark, about 10 g per 15 mL of unsaturated fat for olive oil, as opposed to coconut oil, which contains about 1 g per

15 mL. But when it comes to these healthy unsaturated oils—monounsaturated or polyunsaturated—people simply don't eat enough. The consumption of saturated fats is still too high. A research team in Holland conducted a meta-analysis of sixty clinical trials and found that when polyunsaturated and monounsaturated fats were eaten in place of carbohydrates, bad cholesterol (LDL) levels went down, and the good cholesterol (HDL) increased.[17]

It is well established that some kinds of fats are better than others. Good fats are the unsaturated ones: monounsaturated and polyunsaturated fats. Saturated fats are generally not good for health and are considered bad fats. We know that consuming more saturated fats increases the risk of heart disease and weight gain. However, the connection between saturated fats and obesity has been poorly understood. How come some people can eat all the fat they like and still be skinny? Why don't French women gain weight after eating all those buttery croissants? It turns out that our genes do play a part, and in particular the APOA2 gene influences the effect of saturated fat on weight gain and obesity.[18] The APOA2 gene directs the body to produce a specific protein called apolipoprotein A-II, which enables how the body utilizes different kinds of fat. We will discuss apolipoproteins more in the next section.

As we discussed, unsaturated fats, both monounsaturated and polyunsaturated, may help to decrease the risk of diabetes, cardiovascular diseases, and obesity. The following table lists food sources of monounsaturated and polyunsaturated fats.

Another gene that is implicated in fat metabolism is the FTO gene.[19] The FTO gene gets its name from "fat mass and obesity-associated gene," as this gene determines how successful someone will be at losing weight even after procedures such as bariatric surgery. For people with the AA or TA variant of this FTO gene, a high intake of unsaturated fat and low intake of saturated fat in the diet makes them lose weight faster, decreasing belly fat and the overall risk for obesity.

Food Sources High in Monounsaturated Fat and Polyunsaturated Fat[20]

Sources of Monounsaturated Fat	Monounsaturated Fat (g)
Macadamia nuts, roasted, salted (34 g)	20.1
Hazelnuts, roasted (34 g)	15.6
Almond butter, natural (30 mL)	12.4
Almond nuts, roasted, salted (35 g)	11.8
Olive oil (15 mL))	10.1
Canola oil (15 mL)	8.4

(continued on following page)

Peanut butter, natural (30 mL)	7.8
Flaxseed oil (15 mL)	2.5
Sources of Polyunsaturated Fat	**Polyunsaturated Fat (g)**
Walnuts, dried (25 g)	12.0
Flaxseed oil (15 mL)	9.9
Grapeseed oil (15 mL)	9.6
Sunflower oil (15 mL)	9.1
Soybean oil (15 mL)	8.0
Peanut butter, natural (30 mL)	4.9
Almonds, roasted, salted (35 g)	4.4
Almond butter, natural (30 mL)	4.0

When it comes to cholesterol, why do we need cholesterol at all? Cholesterol is essentially a fatty molecule in our cell membranes and a precursor to some of our hormones. If we don't get enough cholesterol in our food, the liver can also produce it. Cholesterol is needed to build cell membranes and nerve sheaths (i.e., the coverings of our cells). It is also involved in blood clotting and inflammation. We hear about good (HDL) and bad (LDL) cholesterol, but let's examine this in more detail.

HDL Cholesterol

What is high-density lipoprotein (HDL) cholesterol? Cholesterol is transported in our bloodstreams by lipoproteins that act as helper proteins called apolipoproteins. HDL therefore contains cholesterol, triglycerides, and apolipoproteins—with the main one being Apo-AI, which activates an enzyme lecithin–cholesterol acyltransferase (LCAT). This LCAT esterifies cholesterol into a form that can be carried out of blood and tissues more effectively. High density has to do with the fact that this version of lipoprotein contains almost as much protein as fat. This blob of HDL cholesterol is surrounded with lipoprotein, and the 50 percent protein content makes it heavier for its size, and hence the name HDL.

HDL cholesterol is produced in the liver and to a lesser extent by our intestines. Because of its structure and apoproteins, HDL acts as a scavenger by collecting extra cholesterol in different tissues and taking it back to the liver, thereby reducing the risk of arterial disease called by additional cholesterol buildup. We know that endothelial (inside wall) damage to arteries leads to plaque formation, and along with its role as a scavenger, HDL appears to help scrub these walls clean.

Furthermore, most cells accumulate cholesterol and use it in their metabolism but do not have a catabolism (i.e., a mechanism to destroy unused cholesterol). Therefore, they need it transported back to the liver whence it came from in the first place. The LCAT we discussed earlier incorporates this free cholesterol from tissues into the HDL particle, and this eventually helps the uptake of this excess cholesterol by the liver. One of the ways in which this LCAT accomplishes this task of transportation is by using a cholesterol ester transfer protein (CETP). This CETP exchanges the cholesterol esters in the core of HDL cholesterol to apoprotein (Apo-B) containing particles, very low-density lipoprotein (VLDL), and low-density lipoprotein (LDL), and in exchange, it receives triglycerides. Fat-dissolving enzymes in the liver, hepatic lipases, can break down the triglyceride-rich HDL, resulting in smaller-sized HDL particles. These small HDL particles release their Apo-AI, which is degraded by the liver and removed by the kidneys. The CETP pathway results in both the transfer of cholesterol in HDL to the liver and the taking of HDL out of the blood circulation. Therefore, via all these cleanup mechanisms, HDL appears to have a protective effect and hence is often called the "good" cholesterol.

We know that not exercising enough, smoking, and being overweight can raise HDL levels. Also, in diseases like type 2 diabetes, triglyceride levels are often high, and because exchange of cholesteryl esters in HDL particles for triglycerides occurs, the number of triglyceride-rich lipoproteins is increased, resulting in lower HDL cholesterol levels. It is accepted that HDL cholesterol levels greater than 60 milligrams per deciliter (mg/dL) are good and levels under 40 mg/dL are low and therefore not desirable. However, recent research has shown that—as in life choices—too much of a good thing may end up with bad outcomes. A 2021 study done on medications that inhibit CETP pathways showed that they produce substantial increases in HDL cholesterol levels, but these did not translate into lowered cardiovascular risk.[21] Some medications, such as torcetrapib, increased HDL-C by 125 percent and ApoA1 by 46 percent, yet did not reduce cardiovascular events.[22] Worryingly, a study from 2022 in the *Journal of the American Medical Association (JAMA)* looked at very high HDL levels (i.e., those greater than 80 mg/dL). In this cohort study of nearly twenty thousand individuals in the UK and US, those with HDL cholesterol levels greater than 80 mg/dL had a 96 percent higher risk of all-cause mortality and a 71 percent higher risk of cardiovascular mortality.[23] This was staggering. Previously, drugs were being developed to increase HDL levels, but it turns out that beyond a certain level, the results become paradoxical. This higher cardiovascular mortality risk within people with levels greater than 80 mg/dL was more prominent among participants younger than sixty-five years of age.[24] Alcohol could be a factor, as alcohol is known to affect HDL and CETP, although there appear to be specific genes involved.[25] But even accounting for alcohol intake, it appears that the results were the same. The thinking now is that HDL functions as an inflammatory marker and ends up causing more inflammation under certain circumstances, such as increased oxidative stress. Studies have shown that low HDL cholesterol levels predict the risk of infection and autoimmune diseases. Individuals with extremely high HDL cholesterol levels are at increased risk of infectious diseases.[26] One theory is that if high HDL levels are too high, they become less effective at scavenging the LDL cholesterol from arteries. This risk is higher in individuals with certain gene types. In a study of over fifty thousand people, a gene called SCARB1 P376L was associated with heart disease. SCARB1 codes for a major HDL receptor on liver cells, which is a scavenger receptor.[27] Therefore, LDL cholesterol builds up in blood vessel walls, causing plaques that narrow our arteries, leading to heart attacks or strokes.

There are also other genes involved. The hepatic lipase gene, also known as LIPC, encodes an enzyme that plays a key role in blood lipid metabolism. LIPC helps transport HDL cholesterol to the liver, where the processing of cholesterol takes place. Large studies conducted in both men and women show that a genetic variant in LIPC impacts the way HDL cholesterol levels increase in response to physical activity.[28] Generally, individuals who are physically active tend to have higher HDL cholesterol concentrations than those who are sedentary. However, even among those who are physically active, individuals who carry the TT or CT variant in the LIPC gene display an enhanced HDL-raising response when engaging in physical activity, resulting in higher HDL cholesterol than is in individuals without this variant.

More and more, research is revealing our genetic blueprint determines our vulnerability to how our body handles fat and exercise. Another genetic study was the Look AHEAD trial where researchers wanted to study the effect of specific genetic variations on the response to lifestyle interventions targeting dyslipidaemia (abnormal lipid levels) in individuals with obesity and type 2 diabetes.[29] Researchers looked at genetic variations in people with these two conditions and divided them into two groups: one received intensive lifestyle intervention (ILI) and the other, diabetes support and education (DSE). ILI produced greater improvements in HDL cholesterol and triglyceride levels compared to DSE after one year of follow-up.[30] One particular gene variant (CETP rs3764261) strongly influenced baseline HDL levels and actually predicted the response to healthy lifestyle interventions. Women who carried both major alleles—CC variant—of this gene did not show a significant HDL response to the lifestyle intervention, suggesting that this genetic variant was somehow causing a resistance to improvement. And three different LIPC gene variants also determined the HDL response to treatment, with one variant (LIPC-514(C/T) polymorphism, rs1800588) showing a significant increase in HDL levels response to intensive lifestyle intervention but not to diabetes education. In this study, weight loss and improved fitness, the standard treatment recommendations for obese patients with type 2 diabetes mellitus, were studied, but effectiveness of such behavioral therapy was some-what determined by people's genetic profiles.

Therefore, knowing someone's genetic subtypes helps us in recommending specific actions and that is what this book, and my gene-testing program, is about.

In previous sections, we discussed polyunsaturated fatty acids. It turns out that a gene involved in the metabolism of these polyunsaturated fatty acids can adversely affect the levels of HDL cholesterol when dietary omega-6 LA intake is too high or the ratio of omega-6 LA to omega-3 ALA is too high.[31]

Food Sources High in Omega-3 and Omega-6 Fats[32]

Sources	Omega-3 (ALA) (g)	Omega-6 (LA) (g)
Walnuts, English or Persian, dried, pieces (50.7 g)	4.61	19.32
Wheat germ oil (15 mL)	0.95	7.55
Flax seed oil (15 mL)	7.38	1.97
Sardines, Atlantic, canned in oil, drained solids with bone (100 g)	1.46	3.54
Salmon, Atlantic, farmed, baked or broiled (100 g)	2.61	1.93

Sunflower seed kernels, dried (19.4 g)	0.02	4.48
Canola oil (15 mL)	1.30	2.70
Tahini, sesame butter, roasted and toasted kernels (15 mL)	0.06	3.52
Flaxseeds (linseed), whole and ground (10.7 g)	2.46	0.68
Chia seeds, dried (10.8 g)	1.90	0.62
Sunflower oil, oleic (70% and over) (15 mL)	0.03	0.51

We now know that genetic variants in the FADS region are major genetic modifiers that can regulate fatty acid metabolism and epigenetics.[33] The FADS1 gene directs the production of an enzyme called fatty acid desaturase 1. This enzyme converts omega-6 LA and omega-3 ALA to longer-chain polyunsaturated fatty acids that participate in inflammatory and immune systems. Studies show that dietary in-takes of linoleic acid (linoleic acid sources are vegetable oils such as soybean oil, safflower oil, corn oil along with nuts, seeds, and meats) may modulate the impact of the FADS gene on HDL-cholesterol concentration, waist circumference, and BMI. It appears that the C allele was significantly associated with high HDL-cholesterol concentrations in the group with a high intake of PUFAs. Compared to those with the TT variant, individuals who possess the C—either the CC or CT variant of this gene—have lower levels of HDL cholesterol when consumption of omega-6 LA is high. Among those with the CC or CT variant, increasing the proportion of dietary omega-3 ALA to omega-6 LA promotes higher levels of HDL cholesterol.[34]

The Ugliness of Trans Fats

> As I tell patients, while trans fats increase the shelf life of foods, they reduce the shelf life of people.
>
> —Beatrice A. Golomb, MD

As we have discussed, fat is a good source of energy as it produces more calories when compared to proteins or carbohydrates. Fatty acids are also involved in developing cell membranes, nerve sheaths, and blood-clotting factors. As a skin doctor, I know that glycerol is a great moisturiser as it preserves the skin's oily lipid layer. Glycerol is effectively the backbone of a fatty acid. If one considers a lipid molecule, it consists of both glycerol and fatty acids. Glycerol is an alcohol with three carbons, five hydrogens, and three hydroxyl (OH) groups. Fatty acids have a long chain of hydrocarbons with a carboxyl group attached and contain anywhere from four to thirty-six carbons.

We spoke of the health benefits of monounsaturated oils such as olive oil. Monounsaturated fats are typically liquid at room temperatures that become solidified when refrigerated. "Mono" refers to the fact that they have only one carbon-to-carbon double bond (-C=C-). It means that these fats have only one unsaturated double bond (notably of the cis type) in the fatty acid chain, with all the rest being single bonds. Polyunsaturated fatty acids have two or more double bonds in their carbon chain, but again of the cis type. Cis in chemistry means "same side" groups placed on the same side of a double bond (i.e., all the hydrogens on one side for example).

Saturated fats are typically solid at room temperature—think of animal fats such as butter—and become liquid on heating. "Saturated" refers to these fats being saturated with hydrogen molecules, and therefore they have no double bonds between carbon molecules.

Trans fats, as the name indicates, are the opposite of cis. Trans refers to the fatty acid molecules featuring on opposite sides of double bonds. Bacteria in the guts of ruminant animals such as cows produce trans fats but in small quantities. The main source of trans fats is not natural but artificial. For example, industrial methods add additional hydrogen to liquid vegetable oils that contain unsaturated fats to make them more butter-like and solid. Margarine is a classic example and contains elaidic acid,[35] as do deep-fried fast foods and packaged baked goods.[36] French fries, frozen pizza, and microwave popcorn are other examples of fast or processed foods containing trans fats.

Sadly, when it comes to health risks, trans fats are plain ugly, as I will explain in the next sections. We know that the main cholesterol-raising effects of saturated fats is due to the length of the carbon chain. For example, palm oil, coconut oil, and milk fat are denoted as C16:0 (palmitic acid) and, we know, raise cholesterol levels. Stearic acid (C18:0) is typically considered neutral, but eating more cocoa fats from dark chocolate (C18:0) appears to be beneficial. But in fatty acids of the same length, industrial trans fatty acids seem particularly bad. For example, a study was done on elaidic acid, a well-known trans fatty acid, that showed that dietary trans fat 18:1 (elaidic acid) specifically had a detrimental effect when compared to other saturated fats. These results confirm that trans fats are uniquely bad for our lipid profiles. A striking difference between the effects of saturated and trans fatty acids on human lipoprotein metabolism was noted in the study; saturated fats tend to increase both good and bad cholesterol, whereas trans fatty acids depress HDL and increase LDL levels for the worst effect on our cholesterol ratios when compared to all other fats.[37]

Aging has long been associated with DNA methylation, not only in humans but also in smaller animals. I posed the question in a book I cowrote, *The Last Natural Man*[38]: Is aging a disease? This is because aging can be caused or worsened by numerous complex and interacting factors. Oxidative DNA damage, reduction of reproducing stem cells, mitochondrial and nuclear genome mutations, and shortening of telomeres are all implicated in the aging process.[39]

One of the most accurate ways we can measure our biological age is by measuring DNA methylation (DNAm).

More recently, a specifically developed "biological clock," the DNAmGrimAge, outperformed previous DNA clocks in predicting not only lifespan (longevity) but many pathological conditions and diseases (healthspan). This study also showed that specific diet and exercises reduced biomarkers for aging and made a person look, behave, and feel younger. For example, weight gain and obesity was associated with acceleration of aging, and higher consumption of red meat also led to higher DNA methylation levels.[40] Trans fats such as elaidic acid have been shown—in both cell cultures and animal studies—to cause DNA hypermethylation that makes one's biological age older.[41] Therefore, eating fast foods containing trans fats can make you biologically older. Another study, of women, showed that industrial trans fatty acids reduce the success of weight loss when that is a goal. Women wanting to lose weight are better off avoiding highly processed foods, the main source of industrially produced trans fatty acids. While this seems to be common sense, studies showed that doubling elaidic acid blood levels in women was associated with decreased weight loss.[42] We know that as we get older, we develop more cancers because in general more defects occur in our cellular DNA replication. Meta-analyses looking at different cancer types noted that total trans fat intake showed a significant positive association for prostate cancer (with an odds ratio [OR] of 1.49, which means a 49 percent increase in the odds of getting the disease if you are exposed) and colorectal cancer (OR of 1.26, or 26 percent increased odds by consuming more trans fats).[43]

When it comes to health, trans fatty acids are plain ugly. Trans fatty acids found in processed foods in America have been thought to be responsible for thousands of premature deaths from heart attacks each year, with one report from the Pan American Health Association suggesting that 537,000 deaths from coronary heart disease were attributable to trans fat consumption. Of these deaths, 160,000 occurred in the Region of the Americas, 45 percent prematurely.[44] Even when compared to other saturated fats, trans fats reduced HDL (good cholesterol) and increased the ratio of total cholesterol to HDL. And research papers suggest that women with elevated serum levels of trans fatty acid have double the risk of developing breast cancer as compared to women with the lower levels, and also a higher risk of pregnancy-associated complications such as premature births and preeclampsia.[45] The problem is all to do with the hydrogenation of vegetable oils to produce trans fats. The influential Nurses Health Study estimated that a reduction in trans fatty acid intake of 2 percent could reduce the incidence of type 2 diabetes by 40 percent if the fats containing the trans fatty acids were consumed in their original non-hydrogenated form.[46] The list goes on—asthma, allergies and many other illnesses are aggravated by trans fats. If you think these lists are difficult to remember, eating trans fats will make your memory even worse! A study—published by the American Academy of Neurology—conducted by monitoring over 1,600 Japanese citizens older than 60 for a decade, showed that higher serum elaidic acid levels from trans fats were significantly associated with greater risk of developing all-cause dementia.[47]

LAW 18

Trans fats in the diet (found in foods like microwave popcorn, margarine-like spreads, and frozen pizza) can help speed up our biological clocks and therefore worsen the risk of aging and some cancers.

The Dalda Vanaspati Story

The purity of Dalda brings out the natural taste of your food.
—Hindustan Unilever

I was born in England, and my parents moved us to India, and I later moved to New Zealand. As a child in India, every kitchen had a large yellow tin of Dalda with an iconic palm tree logo—so much so that I assumed that Dalda was an Indian word. It turned out it was a case of marketing genius by an originally Dutch company.

Traditionally on the Indian subcontinent, people used ghee (clarified butter) or coconut oil. Ghee is essentially melted butter with the milk solids removed; it is the remaining liquid fat. But ghee was expensive on the Indian subcontinent, where large sections of the populace lived below the poverty line. Traders from Holland had begun selling cheaper hydrogenated highly saturated vegetable oils as an alternative and this led to Dalda. The name was derived from Dada, the original Dutch company, and the *l* in the middle was for Lever Bros (later known as the Hindustan Unilever Corporation). Vanaspati in ancient Indian medial treatises refers to trees that bear fruit but not flowers, although after the Dalda story, it usually means hydrogenated vegetable fats.

Dalda was basically hydrogenated (highly saturated) vegetable fat/oil, vanaspati in common Indian subcontinent terminology. It proved a highly successful and profitable industry, even if was full of trans fats. The aggressive and innovative marketing behind Dalda is the stuff of marketing school legend. In the past, in remote villages, wandering storytellers were roped in to talk about Dalda. The idea was to promote Dalda as a better and "lighter" alternative to clarified butter. In 2015, the marketing even took on religious connotations with Dalda featured everywhere at the Ratha Yatra—the festival held at the city of Puri, in the Indian state of Odisha, and associated with the deity Jagannath—attended by over a million people. In a marketing campaign for Dalda at this religious gathering, the brand was visible on handheld fans, helium balloons, sand art, and even as containers for the pooja ritual ingredients![48] The problem is Dalda was full of trans fats (even if recent moves are being made to reduce this). A report from Outlook India noted:

"Indian snacks contain between 6-30% of TFA (trans fatty acids), far exceeding the safe limit of 2 per cent of total fatty acids."[49] A World Health Organization report on the topic noted a survey of street food in Delhi and Haryana that had found that "25% of snack foods had levels of TFA exceeding the legal limit set by Denmark."[50]

Consumption of such trans fats from processed snacks and deep-fried foods cooked in vanaspati in India are a major health problem. Recently, when the matter was discussed in the lower house of India's parliament, Union Health Minister Mansukh Mandaviya said in a reply to a parliamentary question that "5,400,000 deaths are attributed annually to the consumption of industrially produced trans fats," with an increased "risk of death from any cause of 34%."[51] Manufacturers may be scrambling to say that they are reducing trans fat content, but in general, I would stay clear of foods containing hydrogenated oils.

LAW 19

Trans fats found in vanaspati (hydrogenated cooking oils), widely used in fried foods and snacks, are harmful for health and increase death rates from all causes by a third.

Biohacking Your Fat Genes

Monounsaturated Fat

Monounsaturated fats such as those found in olive oil, almonds, and avocados have been associated with reduced risk for heart disease. Monounsaturated fats can help reduce bad (LDL) cholesterol levels and may also help increase good (HDL) cholesterol.

The PPARy2 gene is involved in the formation of fat cells and is mainly found in fat tissue. Because of its involvement in the formation of fat, PPARy2 can impact weight management and body composition. Specifically, individuals who have the GG or GC variant of the gene tend to experience greater weight loss and lose more body fat, compared to those with the CC variant, when they consume a diet high in monounsaturated fats.[52] For those people, it would be advisable to consume more than 50 percent of your total fat intake from monounsaturated fat. In fact, for anyone, this can also be beneficial for overall heart health.

Total Fat

Fat is an essential part of a healthy diet and is needed for the absorption of the fat-soluble vitamins including vitamins A, D, E, and K. Each gram of fat has more than double the number of calories of carbohydrates or protein on a gram-per-gram basis. This makes fat the most energy-dense nutrient and, therefore, the highest in calories. The total amount and types of fats that you consume can affect heart health and body composition. In general, unsaturated fats (e.g., olive oil, macadamia and Brazil nuts, peanut butter) are heart-healthier and better for you than saturated or trans fats (e.g., cheddar cheese, French fries, butter, salami).

The TCF7L2 gene produces a protein called transcription factor-7 like 2. This protein affects how the body turns on or off a number of other genes. The TCF7L2 gene is involved in maintaining your body weight and composition. Research shows that for individuals who possess the TT variant, the amount of fat in the diet can significantly impact lean/muscle mass versus fat mass as well as increase the risk for being overweight or obese. Furthermore, possessing the TT variant puts you at an increased risk for insulin resistance (reduced ability to control blood sugars) when your total fat intake is high and also increases risk of diabetes in pregnancy.[53] It is therefore recommended that individuals with the TT variant should consume a low-to-moderate fat intake to help achieve weight loss and improve blood sugar glucose levels. For those with the CC or TC variant, there is no difference in weight loss based on the amount of fat consumed, although lower total energy intakes are needed to create a calorie deficit for weight loss.[54]

As the evidence shows, if you possess the CC or TC variant of the TCF7L2 gene, you do not have the same risk of insulin resistance and the amount of fat you consume has no impact on weight loss. However, you should bear in mind that fat has more than double the number of calories on a gram-per-gram basis than carbs or proteins. Therefore, to help ensure that you are consuming a healthy, well-balanced diet, ideally your fat intake should not exceed a third of your total daily energy intake as part of an energy-restricted diet.

Food Sources High in Total Fat[55]

Sources of Total Fat	Amount (g)
Macadamia nuts, roasted, salted (34 g)	26
Cheddar cheese (50 g)	17
Olive oil (15 mL)	14
Swiss cheese (50 g)	14
Pistachios, shelled, roasted, salted (31 g)	14
Ground beef, lean, crumbled, pan-fried (75 g)	11
Goat cheese (50 g)	11
Bacon, pork, broiled, pan-fried, or roasted (24 g)	10

Salmon, sockeye, baked or broiled (75 g)	8
Butter (5 g)	4

5

Eat for Your Gene Type

A new scientific truth does not triumph by convincing its opponents and making them see the light, but rather because its opponents eventually die, and a new generation grows up that is familiar with it.

—Max Planck

John Yudkin's Story

In the 1970s, John Yudkin was a noted physiologist and nutritionist and was a founding professor of the Department of Nutrition at Queen Elizabeth College, London, no less. He wrote a book, *Pure, White, and Deadly*, about the dangers of sugar.[1] Yudkin was concerned that the establishment was barking up the wrong tree in blaming only animal fats for the

alarming rise in coronary disease. In his view, the real culprit
was sugar, especially sucrose, which is essentially a combination of glucose and fructose. Yudkin had been concerned
about industrialized diets and increase in sugar intake for over
two decades. In 1964, he wrote an article suggesting sugar was
responsible for diabetes, heart disease, dental cavities, and
obesity. Yudkin felt that consumption of animal fats had been
a part of human history so was part of man's genetic makeup,
and modern man was substituting sugars for protein from animal fats and other nutrition from vegetables. As Yudkin wrote
in a 1964 article for *Proceedings of the Nutrition Society*,

> It is generally held that, for the greater part of the million or more
> years of his existence, man was a hunter and forager; his diet was
> largely the bodies of animals he killed or found as carrion, with
> relatively small amounts of leaves, fruits, and roots. Being omnivo-
> rous, he could of course sustain himself, if necessary, with a lower
> proportion of meat, and a higher proportion of vegetable foods,
> but by and large his diet was relatively poor in carbohydrate. . . .[2]

Yudkin then went to analyze the diets of different populations around the world.

> I have made calculations for the nine low-income countries, Brazil,
> Ceylon, Chile, Egypt, Greece, India, Pakistan, Philippines, and Yugo-
> slavia, with a total population of some 650 million. Compared
> with the pre-war period, the average calorie intake in 1958 had

increased by 9%, but meat consumption had fallen by 9% and animal protein intake by 7%. At the same time, sugar consumption had increased by 105%. . . .[3]

Yudkin also compared and contrasted his findings between less-affluent countries and Western economies with higher incomes.

In the wealthier countries, the intake of highly palatable sweetened food and drinks, of which the sugar alone contributes over 500 kcal per head a day, is undoubtedly a potent contribution to the high prevalence of obesity, both in adults and in children. . . . Sugar may specifically be a factor in the causation of other diseases. Amongst these, I include dental caries, diabetes mellitus, dyspepsia and peptic ulceration, and myocardial infarction.[4]

Much to the delight of big food corporations, a prominent American physiologist, Ancel Keys, rubbished Yudkin when he wrote: "The widely publicized theory that sucrose in the diet is a major factor in the development of coronary heart disease has been examined. The theory is not supported by acceptable clinical, epidemiological, theoretical, or experimental evidence."[5]

Yudkin, while he continued to write articles in the popular press, never received recognition for his theories during his lifetime. Almost fourteen years after Yudkin's death, Robert Lustig, a pediatric endocrinologist, became known for calling fructose sugar a poison that was responsible for America's obesity epidemic. In a YouTube video[6] that has been watched by over twenty million people, Lustig explained what he believes is really making humans obese.

Lustig may be nutrition's philosopher-activist who plumbs the failure of humans in eating artificially enhanced sugars based on corporate promises and medicine's willful blindness. In his talk, Lustig pointed out that both the Japanese and the Atkins diets have been considered beneficial, yet they are polar opposites: the former is full of carbs while the latter is heavy in fats. The commonality between these diets is the reduction of sugar, especially high amounts of fructose.

Lustig noted that before 1975, we had never consumed high fructose corn syrup. He estimated each person is now consuming sixty-three pounds (28.5 kg) of corn syrup per year. Lustig was particularly keen to distinguish the chemistry of high fructose corn syrup: one glucose and one fructose. Glucose has a six-membered ring, and fructose has a five-membered ring. "They are not the same," he said, "Believe me, they're not the same."[7]

Lustig went on to discuss how when glucose and fructose are linked together, they form sucrose, which is what we call table sugar. Lustig concluded this topic with a flourish, saying "We have this enzyme in our gut called sucrase—it kills that bond in two seconds flat, and you absorb it. Basically, high fructose corn syrup [and] sucrose—it's a non-issue, it's a wash. They are the same."[8]

So, interestingly, Lustig—who probably never heard of Yudkin as he has never referenced him that I've seen—essentially reached the same conclusions about the societal scourge of sugar. But now times have changed. The dangers of sugar are increasingly spoken about, even in political circles. In 2018, the British government introduced a "sugar tax" (i.e., a levy on soft drinks containing added sugar).[9] Around the same time, I was invited to speak at Chatham House, London. In my talk titled "Germs, Genes and Geography," essentially about understanding and biohacking our genes, I pointed out the anomalies and loopholes that food businesses had exploited.[10] For example, in a nod to the benefits of milk, milkshakes and smoothies were exempt from the sugar tax, although I pointed out in my lecture that they were just as sweet as other sugar products.

Recently, research has focused on answering the question about the dangers of sugars: Is it only the type of sugar or also the quantity? A large study published in *BMC Medicine* looked to address the associations between types and sources of dietary carbohydrates and cardiovascular disease (CVD) incidence.[11] Over 100,000 UK Biobank participants (aged thirty-seven to seventy-three) who were free from cardiovascular disease and diabetes at baseline were included and followed up for almost ten years. Free sugar intake (i.e., sugars in processed foods and drinks) was measured; natural fruit and vegetable sugars were excluded. The most common forms of sugar the study participants ate were cookies, cakes, fruit juice, sugar-sweetened beverages, and desserts.[12] What this UK study found was that higher free sugar intake was associated with higher CVD incidence and higher triglyceride concentrations within all lipoproteins. Based on this, I estimate that if a 5 percent increase in the share of a person's total energy intake came from free sugars, then that person could experience a 6 percent higher risk of heart disease and a 10 percent higher risk of stroke. It is noteworthy that American guidelines still suggest that added sugars should make up no more than 10 percent of one's daily calories, not lower, as it should be.[13]

The problem appears to be when one consumes almost equal portions of fructose and glucose. Sucrose has a 50 percent fructose and 50 percent glucose split, and high fructose corn syrup in sodas is usually 55 percent fructose to 45 percent glucose.[14] Honey, in contrast, has a 45/35 split, with the rest containing maltose, sucrose, and other complex carbohydrates.[15] Honey was the only added sugar in prehistoric times and accounted for 2 to 3 percent of energy intake.[16] Therefore, one can see where we are getting things wrong.

LAW 20

Added sugars—sucrose and high fructose corn syrup—found in processed foods such as candy and sweet drinks increase your risk of heart disease and strokes. It is best to have natural fruit sugar or honey and ensure

that only around 5 percent of your energy intake comes
from added sugars.

The Problem with Artificial Sweeteners

Respect your body and look forward to feeling healthy and
clean. Your body deserves better than laboratory-made
sweetness.

—Damon Gameau

With the adverse publicity surrounding sugar, processed
food manufacturers turned to artificial sweeteners like
aspartame (Nutrasweet or Equal found in fizzy drinks such
as Coke Zero and even chewing gum), sucralose (Splenda),
or acesulfame potassium (Sweet One or Sunett). And more
recently, erythritol (from fermented corn) and Stevia (from
Stevia plant leaves) have been used as artificial sweeteners. In
theory, using artificial sweeteners as sugar substitutes appear
plausible. But industry does not reckon with the power of the
human brain or the brain-gut and brain-skin connections.
If we taste something and it tastes sweet to us, our brain
sends the same messages as it would when we taste sugar.
Therefore the response of the gastrointestinal system is
the same: insulin is secreted in response to artificial sweeteners. And studies have confirmed that as insulin levels
rise in the blood in response to these artificial sweeteners,

we eventually become insulin resistant and can end up with diabetes.[17]

It therefore transpires that artificial sweeteners—rather like fake news—is no good for us. But the story gets worse. A population cohort study in France followed over 100,000 people, mostly females in their forties and fifties, for twelve years (2009–2021) and found a direct association between higher artificial sweetener consumption (especially aspartame, acesulfame potassium, and sucralose) and increased cardiovascular disease risk. This study, published in the *British Medical Journal* (*BMJ*), concluded that such sweeteners might represent a modifiable risk factor for cardiovascular disease prevention and should not be considered a healthy and safe alternative to sugar.[18] Aspartame was recently added to a list of potential carcinogens by the WHO, although the evidence for this is, at present, limited.[19] In a similar vein, many randomized trials have shown that artificial sweeteners do increase the risk of metabolic syndrome.[20] Artificial sweeteners and sugary drinks not only increased the risk of type 2 diabetes and cardiovascular disease but they also increased all-cause mortality.[21] This may be because of metabolic effects and also alterations in gut microbiomes. Even newer artificial sweeteners are not exempt. As reported in *Nature Medicine*, erythritol, a "sugar alcohol," has been found to increase blood clots and thrombotic diseases.[22] Stevia, from the Stevia rebaudiana plant, was considered relatively safe, but increasingly there are reports about potential endocrine and metabolic dysfunction, and alterations in the gut microbiome with unknown long-term effects.[23]

LAW 21

Artificial sweeteners used in candy and drinks also increase the risk of diabetes, cardiovascular diseases, and thrombotic events and are best avoided. Aspartame is a potentially cancer-causing agent, and Stevia alters the microbiome of the gut adversely.

Biohacking Your Sugar Genes

Sugar and Aging: Advanced Glycation End Products (AGEs)

As we age, sugar molecules from the foods we eat build up inside our body and stick to proteins and lipids, affecting their function. These sugar-bound complexes are called advanced glycation end products (AGEs). In the skin, sugars bind to collagen and elastin, which are important dermal structural components. This makes both collagen and elastin brittle and prone to breaking, which leads to a more wrinkled, saggy skin appearance. While this process occurs naturally over time, eating too much sugar, as well as exposure to UV rays, may also accelerate skin glycation.[24]

Other sources of AGEs are foods browned or prepared at high temperatures, such as donuts, barbequed meats, and caramel-colored soft drinks. These AGEs promote oxidation and inflammation, and they damage not only the skin but tissues throughout the body. The enzyme glyoxalase 1 (GLO1) is involved in the body's defence mechanism against AGEs. Research shows that variation in the GLO1 gene affects the enzyme's activity, which may make some individuals more susceptible to the skin-aging effects of AGEs. Research on GLO1 has found that two variants of this specific gene affect the resulting enzyme's activity in the blood. Individuals can carry zero to four copies of the risk variants, and GLO1 activity decreases proportionally with each additional risk variant.[25] Individuals who carry more risk variants may be less efficient at neutralising AGEs, and the resulting glycation damage could lead to fine lines, wrinkles, and sagging skin. The glyoxalase system, mediated by this GLO1, has a protective effect against formation of AGEs. Impairment of this enzymatic activity leads to a higher risk of a multitude of age-related-diseases such as Alzheimer's disease, Parkinson's disease, and cancer.[26]

I originally became interested in AGEs because they make our skin age faster. Many medical researchers have studied blood sugar levels and the impact of stress. One study from Germany found that during stressful examinations, HbA1c (blood glucose levels) increased significantly in healthy medical students which reverted to normal after a few months.[27] These findings were noted in healthy, nondiabetic individuals, yet psychological stress increased glycation, and therefore, prolonged stress can possibly increase your risk of diabetes. Glycation, when due to stress as opposed to diet, is also at play in how quickly we appear to age. Glycation in skin reduces elasticity and increases wrinkles, as AGEs bind to collagen protein.

For people with higher sugar intake, diabetes, or high stress, the skin elasticity curve shifts downward, confirming that glycation stress is a major factor in the reduction of skin elasticity (i.e., making your skin saggy).

If your genetic profile suggests that you are at a higher risk of glycation, it is important for you to reduce sugar intake, reduce stress (by practicing meditation or yoga, for example), and increase muscular exercise to help your skin look younger. Muscle load or weight training is particularly important as well, as more than 80 percent of blood glucose is consumed in skeletal muscle, and the more muscle one maintains, the less insulin resistance—if tissue becomes less resistant to insulin, cells can break down sugar better using insulin, thereby leading to less glycation end products.[28] In fact, this research into glycation led to my skin research lab, Healthy Skin Lab, creating a range of skin products designed to reduce wrinkling of skin and the effects of aging.

Glycemic Index (GI)

The glycemic index (GI) of any food indicates the rate at which the carbohydrate in that food is broken down into glucose and absorbed from the gut into the blood. In high GI foods, this occurs quickly, causing your blood glucose (sugar) level to rise rapidly. In low GI foods, carbohydrate is digested slowly, resulting in a more gradual rise in blood glucose levels. Therefore, low GI foods are inherently preferable.

Starch basically contains amylose (which makes up about 20 to 30 percent of the starch) and amylopectin (70 to 80 percent)[29]—the former is soluble, while starches like rice, with high amylopectin content, become sticky when cooked. The lower the amylose, the higher the GI index. Not all starches are bad. An example of this is brown rice, which is high in resistant starch and has been shown to reduce both blood sugars and triglycerides.

As a skin doctor, I often talk about skin cancer, especially my preference for cleansers being pH-neutral. This means that these products must have the same pH as skin, which is acidic with a pH of around 5.5. As humans reach puberty, our skin becomes acidic, probably to inhibit bacterial colonization. Soaps, as we know, are alkaline with a pH of 7 to 9 and disrupt the skin barrier and affect the skin microbiome, making people prone to dermatitis and skin irritations.

When it comes to our guts, the stomach is extremely acidic due to the need to break down foods and has a pH that ranges from 1 to 2.5. The pH rises to 6.6 to 7.5 in the small and the large intestine (i.e., progressively rises from 5.5–7.0 in the small bowel to 6.5–7.5 in the distal ileum).

If we consider breads, sourdough breads have pH levels that typically fall between 3.5 and 5.5, making them mildly acidic, whereas other breads have a pH of 5 to 6.5. The more acidic the bread, the lower the glycemic index (GI). The higher the glycemic index, the more the food causes higher sugar levels in the body, and therefore low GI foods are preferable. Similarly, the higher the fiber content of the food, such as brown rice or quinoa, the lower the glycemic index. This is because increasing fiber, or the acidity, slows the rate of digestion, resulting in a lower GI.

Some people with variants of the TCF7L2 gene have an inherently higher risk of developing type 2 diabetes if they consume high GI foods. Research shows that American women with the high-risk GT or TT variant of the gene are at greater risk of developing type 2 diabetes, so they are better off consuming more whole grains.[30]

Evolutionary biology is also something to consider, as your ancestral diets can shape your starch-digestion genes. If your ancestors ate high-starch diets, you are more likely to have the TT or AT variant of the AMY1 gene; if they consumed lower starch diets, you may end up with the AA variant of the AMY1 gene and find it difficult to digest starch. A study done on Korean men found that individuals who have the AA variant of the AMY1 gene have a decreased ability to break down starch and a greater risk for insulin resistance when consuming a high-starch diet.[31]

Not all carbohydrates are bad. Indeed, carbohydrates are the main source of energy for our brain and working muscles, so this discussion is not meant to scare you away from consuming carbohydrates completely. There are three main types of carbohydrates: sugar, starch, and fiber. Healthful sources of carbohydrates in the diet include minimally processed starches such as whole grain breads and cereals, rice, root vegetables, beans, lentils, chickpeas, fruits, and low-fat dairy products, when they are consumed in moderation. Unhealthy sources of carbohydrates include refined grains, sugar-sweetened beverages, and certain baked goods. Instead of white breads and baked goods, white rice, and pasta, incorporate more 100 percent whole grains, brown rice, and whole wheat foods.

Sugar Preference

Sugar intake is partly determined by our sweet taste preference and cravings for certain foods and beverages. There is considerable variability in individuals' preferences and cravings for sweet foods and beverages. There are many factors that may impact your preference for sugary foods, including the age that you are first introduced to sweets and psychological associations between consuming these foods and certain life experiences or emotions. In addition to "pleasure-generating" signals in the brain given off in response to eating or drinking something sweet, there are specialized areas in the brain that regulate both food intake and glucose (sugar) levels in the body. Research has shown that your intake of sweet foods can be determined by a genetic variant that regulates blood glucose levels in your body.[32]

Glucose transporter type 2 (GLUT2) is involved in regulating glucose (sugar) in the body. The expression of this gene has been found in areas of the brain that are involved in controlling food intake. Individuals who possess the TT or TC variant of this gene seem to have a greater preference for sweet foods and beverages and are more likely to over consume sugar.[33] In addition, those who have the variant associated with higher sweet food intake, have also been shown to have a higher risk of dental cavities.[34]

High-sugar foods are often disguised in food and drinks we wouldn't typically assume were high in sugar. For example, 1 cup (250 mL) of iced cappuccino has 28 g of sugar; however, 1 cup of citrus juice has 32 g of sugar.[35] The WHO recommends that we derive less than 10 percent of our energy intake from sugar, or less than 5 percent if possible.[36] For an average human, with a normal BMI, that works out to about 25 g of sugar per day. One can of cola or 30 mL of maple syrup means that you've already exceeded your daily sugar limit.

Food Sources High in Sugar[37]

Sources of High-Sugar Foods	Amount (g)
Chocolate milkshake (250 mL)	52
Caramel candies (40 g)	26
Milk chocolate (50 g)	26
Cola (250 mL)	24
Orange juice, frozen, diluted (250 mL)	22
Caramel-coated popcorn (37 g)	20
Jellybeans (28 g)	20
Maple syrup (15 mL)	12
Jams and Preserves (15 mL)	10

Novak Djokovic's Story

Let food be thy medicine and medicine be thy food.

—Hippocrates

Everyone knows Novak Djokovic, the Serbian tennis super-star. Prior to 2010, he was considered a "tanker." At the end of grueling matches, he would run out of steam and hyperventi-late—to the extent that fellow tennis pros like Andy Roddick belittled Djokovic. As an article in *Sports Illustrated* noted: "Roddick was asked about Djokovic's myriad injuries and penchant for calling for medical timeouts. Roddick responded by suggesting that Djokovic was suffering from everything from a common coughing cold to anthrax and SARS. 'If it's there, it's there,' Roddick said."[38]

Fast-forward to thirteen years later, and Novak Djokovic has won more grand slam tennis tournaments than anyone else. And most of his twenty-four slam wins came during the time when Roger Federer and Rafael Nadal were playing; Djokovic has won grueling matches against them more times than anyone else. Roddick won a solitary US open title in 2003.[39] So, what caused the turnaround?

Around 2010, Novak Djokovic met with a Serbian doctor by the name of Igor Cetojevic who diagnosed gluten intoler-ance. Cetojevic's methods may have been unorthodox and not the genetic testing my lab undertakes, but once Djokovic elim-inated gluten from his diet, his fortunes changed. Dramatically. He is now the person who is easier to beat in three-set matches rather than the longer five-set ones at the major events—where he is almost impossible to conquer by men fifteen years younger than him![40]

So what is this gluten? We know gluten is a protein in grains such as wheat, barley, and rye; it is what makes our bread chewy. When I wrote my previous book, *The Genetics of Health*, on the topic of genes and wellness, I mentioned Aretaeus, a physician in Cappadocia almost two thousand years ago. With no lab tests available, he was able to differentiate gluten sensitivity (similar to an allergic reaction) and gluten intolerance causing celiac disease (the full-blown autoimmune disease) just from clinical observation.[41] Until recently—even still today—many in mainstream medicine are sceptical that one can have issues with gluten without being a full celiac. In remote Indigenous tribes, celiac disease is virtually unknown and has only recently been reported in the Coast Salish First Nations population on the west coast of Canada, for example.[42] It is probably due to human being moving onto industrlialized and processed foods.

Celiac disease is the autoimmune condition caused by sensitivity to gluten in wheat. One of the reasons it hasn't been studied as well is because scientists lacked animal models that are often used in medical research. It appears that the Irish setter dog is an exception and is able to develop gluten-related diseases.[43] Being autoimmune means celiac disease can affect multiple systems such as the skin, gut, and bones.[44]

Wheat cultivation methods have been considered the cause in the increase in celiac disease in populations, and we now know that around 1 percent of Western populations have this disease.[45] People with celiac disease require a gluten-free diet for life. Non-celiac gluten sensitivity (NCGS) is a milder form of gluten intolerance that may affect up to 6 percent of the population.[46] Individuals with NCGS often experience diarrhoea, abdominal pain, fatigue, and headaches when they consume gluten-containing foods. This may explain Djokovic's earlier fatigue. Djokovic is now well-known for speaking about his diagnosis of gluten sensitivity in his book, *Serve to Win*, where he talks about the diet that changed his life.[47]

However, these adverse effects of gluten in individuals who do not have celiac disease are poorly understood and NCGS remains controversial. Skin disorders due to gluten sensitivity were first described in modern times by Dr. Louis Duhring of the University of Pennsylvania in 1884 and was named dermatitis herpetiformis as the rash resembled the viral vesicles caused by herpes.[48]

Some people are not convinced about this non-celiac gluten tolerance. These researchers feel that patients are actually reacting to an excess of poorly absorbed carbohydrates present in wheat and many other foods. Those carbohydrates—called FODMAPs, short for fermentable oligosaccharides, disaccharides, monosaccharides, and polyols—can cause bloating when they ferment in the gut and are the real culprits.[49] This has led to the low-FODMAP diet as a trial in people suspected of non-celiac gluten insensitivity.[50]

The HLA genes produce a group of proteins called the human leukocyte antigen complex, which are responsible for how the immune system distinguishes between the body's own proteins and foreign, potentially harmful proteins. Research has shown that the HLA genes are the most important genetic predictor of gluten intolerance.[51] More than 90 percent of people with celiac disease have the DQ2 or DQ8 risk version of HLA, compared to only 30 to 40 percent of the general population.[52] Six variations in the HLA genes can be used to classify individuals into predefined risk groups for gluten intolerance. Risk prediction is based upon a scale of low, medium, or high risk.

Gluten-free foods include all unprocessed vegetables, fruit, dairy products, meat, fish, poultry, nuts, legumes, seeds, fats, and oils. Gluten-free grains include rice, quinoa, corn, buckwheat, amaranth, and millet. For individuals who need to follow a gluten-free diet, foods to avoid include any products that are made with wheat, rye, barley, or triticale. Pure oats should be consumed in moderation if tolerated, while regular oats (which contain wheat) should be avoided. For the vast majority of the population, consuming a gluten-free diet is unnecessary. Processed gluten-free products often have more calories, sodium, added sugar and fat and fewer nutrients compared to their gluten-containing counterparts.

Biohacking Your Gluten Genes

Many scientific journal articles point to skin issues such as skin sensitivity, dermatitis, and psoriasis-like rashes as being due to gluten intolerance, even if you do not have the full-blown celiac disease profile.[53] The theory is that gluten intolerance stimulates your innate immunity and makes it attack your own body and skin. Itching is common, further aggravating skin rashes. In my clinical practice, I have noted gluten intolerance and skin issues more commonly in female patients.

Your gene profile will indicate where you sit on the gluten spectrum. If your risk is high, it is better to completely eliminate gluten from your diet. If your risk is medium, you may be fine with occasionally consuming gluten, or in very small amounts. Being at medium risk for developing celiac disease does not mean you have celiac disease. Speak to a healthcare professional if you experience diarrhea, steatorrhea, cramps, flatulence, fatigue, or joint pain while consuming gluten-containing foods, or if you have a family member with celiac disease. If you do not possess the DQ2 or DQ8 risk genotype, this rules out celiac disease in almost all cases.

Sources of Gluten

Known Sources of Gluten	Hidden Sources of Gluten
Bread	Salad dressing
Pasta	Pudding
Cereal	Crab stick

(continued on following page)

Crackers and chips	Vegan meat substitute
Oats*	Potato chips
Baked goods	French fries
Malt	Soup stock cubes
Soy sauce	Chocolate and candy
Gravy	Processed meat
Barley- or wheat-based beer	Canned soup
Vinegars	Instant rice
Wheat—including rye, spelt, and barley	Ice cream

*Pure oats do not contain gluten; however, oats are often cross-contaminated with gluten-containing grains.

LAW 22

Gluten intolerances are not created equal. Some people have a full blown autoimmune version with severe

health consequences; in some, it can be a gluten sensi-
tivity that can cause gut and energy problems.

Lactose: We Need to Talk about Cow's Milk

Milk is as uniform a liquor as ye chaos was. If beer be poured into it & ye mixture let stand till it be dry, the surface of ye curdled substance will appear as rugged & mountainous as the Earth in any place.

—Sir Isaac Newton

As a skin MD, I have long noted that that cow's milk aggravates conditions such as acne and rosacea. We know that acne is a chronic inflammatory condition in hair follicles, and this can lead to them getting clogged and becoming open comedones (blackheads) or closed comedones (whiteheads). Meta-analyses have shown that any dairy, such as milk, yogurt, and cheese, is associated with an increased incidence of acne, especially in people under the age of thirty.[54]

I began my skin practice in 1996. At that time, the link between consumption of milk (or lactose, in general) and inflammatory skin diseases was not known. In 2005, a retrospective study mentioned earlier asked 47,355 adult women to recall their high school diet. The study was confined to those who had sought physician assistance for acne. This large study found that acne was positively associated with the reported quantity of milk ingested—even skim milk.[55] Why did human beings begin to drink cow's milk in the first place?

It is interesting that until less than ten thousand years ago, the human consumption of cow's milk was unknown. Historically, animal milk consumption originated from our desperation to survive during a famine. Genes are all about propagation of a species and as some people developed genes to digest lactose, these were passed on to future generations.

Drinking animal milk became advantageous, even crucial, to our evolutionary progress throughout history, such as helping us against the threat of deadly diseases like malaria. Even today, malaria causes over half a million deaths a year globally. Studies done on mice today have shown that fermented milk has some antimalarial effect, reducing the risk of infection.[56] The calcium and phosphate content of milk is also beneficial against rickets.[57]

Dairy farming originated in the Middle East and was then adopted in Europe—accordingly, lactose intolerance occurs in about 25 percent of people in Europe; 50 to 80 percent of people of Hispanic origin, south India, and Africa and Ashkenazi Jews; and almost all adults in Asia and Native Americans cannot digest lactose properly.[58] This is because people living in Africa and East and Southeast Asia were mostly hunter-gatherers, leading to a high degree of lactose intolerance in adults. In places with high malaria rates, the ability to digest lactose persisted for longer, indicating the link between lactose genes and diseases.[59]

Recently, I was interested in a study that was done in Sweden on the association between lactose intolerance and cancers, and more specifically breast cancer. This large 2015 cohort study, involving over twenty thousand women, noted that people with lactose intolerance who did not consume dairy products, especially cow's milk, had decreased risks of lung, breast, and ovarian cancers. We know cancers always have a genetic preponderance. What was interesting in this study was that they also studied these women's family members, who did not have this lower risk, and the reduced risk was specifically attributed to these individuals' avoidance of dairy products.[60]

Married scientists Harald zur Hausen and Ethel-Michele de Villiers are based at DKFZ, the German Cancer Research Center in Heidelberg. They believe that viral pathogens cause chronic inflammation, which leads to cancer, and in their studies, they have identified European cows as a potential source. Their team identified viral single-stranded DNA rings, which they have called bovine meat and milk factors (BMMF), in the intestines of patients with colon cancer. They believe that this new class of pathogen deserves to become the focus of cancer development and research into further chronic diseases.[61] Why must one take zur Hausen de Villiers seriously? It is because this was the same man who first postulated that cervical cancer was sexually transmitted due to the HPV virus, and he was ridiculed. In 2008, the Nobel Assembly at Karolinska Institutet awarded the Nobel Prize in Physiology or Medicine to Harald zur Hausen for "for his discovery of human papilloma viruses causing cervical cancer."[62] His new hypothesis is that milk products and bovine proteins harbor viruses that can later lead to breast cancer, multiple sclerosis, and diabetes.[63]

New Zealand, the world's biggest exporter of milk, has very high rates of both breast cancer[64] and multiple sclerosis (MS).[65] MS was particularly interesting. When I lived in India, I had never come across a case, and standard medical teaching was that MS is more prevalent at the poles and rare in the tropics. But Israel, for example, is an outlier, with very high rates of MS even though it is not a polar country.[66] Is it a coincidence that Israel has a high dairy intake?[67] Is zur Hausen correct? Time will tell.

Biohoacking Your Lactose Genes

As I mentioned earlier, lactose intolerance is more common in people of African and Asian descent. Lactose intolerance is controlled by a DNA sequence located within a gene called MCM6.

When we break down lactose, it turns into glucose and galactose (another sugar with the same formula as glucose and fructose: $C_6H_{12}O_6$). Sometimes, when people are ill and their bowel is not functioning normally, they can also temporarily become lactose intolerant. We now know the risky variants of the MCM6 gene that lead to lactose intolerance: CC or CT. If you have the TT variant, you have a low or no risk of being lactose intolerant.[68]

Lactose is a naturally occurring sugar found in dairy products. When lactose is properly digested, it is broken down into two different sugar molecules: glucose and galactose. Lactase is the enzyme needed to break down lactose. Some people do not produce any, or enough, lactase. Because of this, lactose passes through the intestines undigested. When this occurs, gut bacteria in the intestines ferment the lactose, which produces gas that leads to bloating and cramps and causes water to enter the intestine quickly, leading to diarrhea. These are the uncomfortable symptoms associated with lactose intolerance. These symptoms can develop as early as one hour after you consume lactose-containing products. Typically, individuals with lactose intolerance may have to consume a lactose-free or lactose-reduced diet for life or consume dairy products with a meal to reduce the impact of lactose on the gastrointestinal system.

Sometimes you can train your body to produce more lactase enzyme by gradually introducing lactose into your diet. Research shows that individuals who consume a lactose-free diet are at a greater risk of inadequate calcium and vitamin D intake compared to individuals who can tolerate lactose.[69] Calcium and vitamin D are important for building and maintaining strong bones and teeth. If you have lactose intolerance, you can still get enough calcium and vitamin D in the diet through lactose-free milk as well as fortified milk alternatives such as soy and almond beverages. Calcium and vitamin D are not added to all milk alternatives, so be sure to read the label to check that the products you are choosing have been "fortified with calcium and vitamin D."

In my practice, I have noted late-onset acne-like eruptions in women quite commonly, as also noted in many studies.[70] If you are prone to breakouts or skin inflammation, avoid lactose. However, if your gene profile suggests a degree of lactose intolerance, you may find your skin is better if you eliminate it completely from your diet. Goat's milk is associated with inflammation, even if used to make soaps. A study showed that goat's milk soap for the management of inflammatory skin conditions appears to be associated with clinically significant sensitization, and allergy to goat's milk–based foods is also noted.[71]

To help meet your calcium and vitamin D needs, aim to include one serving of dairy, if tolerated, and one to two calcium- and vitamin D-fortified lactose-free milk or dairy alternatives such as soy or almond beverages.

Food Sources High in Lactose[72]

Sources of Lactose	Amount (g)
Regular milk (250 mL)	15.75
Yogurt, natural (200 g)	10.0*

Ricotta cheese (120 g)	2.4
Cream (15 mL)	0.6
Ice cream (100 g)	3.3
Cream cheese (22 g)	0.55

*The lactose content in yogurt decreases each day, even while it sits in the fridge, because the natural bacteria present in yogurt use lactose for energy.

LAW 23

Humans have only consumed milk for less than 10 percent of our existence. As we become older, we develop a degree of lactose intolerance. Lactose intolerance is more common in African and Asian populations. Fermented dairy foods have lower lactose than fresh sources.

Sodium: Salty Science and History

A marine protozoan is an aqueous salty system in an aqueous salty medium, but a man is an aqueous salty system in a medium in which there is but little water and most of that poor in salts.

—John Z. Young

As land mammals, we humans are designed to live outside water. As I mentioned in the section on vitamin D, our cells needed calcium regulators because seawater and land water have different calcium concentrations. The same is true of sodium regulation. Marine creatures have different adaptations to live in seawater that has about 3.5 percent salt by weight.[73] Marine mammals that eat fish are essentially eating food with a salt content similar to that of their own blood, thereby avoiding fluid retention or leakage. They don't consume added salt as we humans do.

We know table salt is chemically sodium chloride. But it is the sodium component that causes blood pressure issues. Why did humans start adding salt to food? This was because around five thousand years ago, civilizations discovered the ability of salt to preserve food and to prevent meat from rotting.[74]

Both human and animal studies show that more sodium makes blood pressure increase.[75] However, because we get most of our sodium from salt, we tend to use these terms interchangeably when discussing blood pressure risk. And studies show that lowering salt reduces blood pressure. For example, there was a natural health survey done in Britain that looked at salt consumption and deaths from strokes and heart attacks. From 2003 to 2011, deaths from strokes and ischaemic heart disease (due to blocked arteries) reduced by 40 percent. During the same period, blood pressure in the population was lowered by around 3 millimeters of mercury (mmHg), and the average person's salt intake went down by 15 percent.[76] This demonstrates that reducing blood pressure even in small amounts by eating less salt can have major health benefits. Following this UK study, the prestigious *New England Journal of Medicine* reported on the projected effect of dietary salt reductions on future cardiovascular disease.[77] They noted:

> Reducing dietary salt by 3 g per day is projected to reduce the annual number of new cases of CHD by 60,000 to 120,000, stroke by 32,000 to 66,000, and myocardial infarction by 54,000 to 99,000 and to reduce the annual number of deaths from any cause by 44,000 to 92,000. All segments of the population would benefit, with blacks benefiting proportionately more, women benefiting particularly from stroke reduction, older adults from reductions in CHD events, and younger adults from lower mortality rates.[78]

What was interesting to me was that segments of the populations benefited differently. One can understand gender differences due to hormonal effects, but why the great disparity between white and Black populations in America? What this means is, our response to salt may be determined by our genetic makeup. This is something we can test for, as I will discuss in the next section.

Professor Graham MacGregor from the Queen Mary University of London has long been a proponent of salt reduction. In a commentary on salt consumption, MacGregor talked about an experiment that was done on chimpanzees. Chimps can weigh up to 50 kg, but usually eat less than 0.5 g of salt a day. When salt in their diet was increased to 15 g a day, their blood pressure rose slowly, and it was still on the rise after one year. The blood pressure eventually returned to normal when salt intake was reduced.[79]

In MacGregor's paper on salt, he discussed the British strategy to make reductions in the salt content of all processed foods by 10 to 25 percent.[80] Interestingly, people cannot taste a reduction of this amount and over time, our taste buds get used to having smaller salt concentrations. The idea is the whole population over time begins to eat less salt.

The things we can control are our own actions and taking responsibility for our health. We know babies need very little salt, less than a gram a day. Research has shown that babies given salty foods develop a lifelong preference for eating more salty food with bad health consequences.[81] In Australia, for example, the National Health and Research Council recommends 200–400 mg of sodium per day for babies 1–3 years old and recommend a limit not exceeding 920 mg of sodium per day in teenagers aged 14–18.[82] American adults eat an average of 3.6 g of salt a day.[83]

Because, as the UK experience showed, we cannot detect if the salt content is decreased by a quarter, it should be simple to do. Why the resistance? It makes these foods less addictive for children. No wonder fast food chains target children in their advertising and offer toys and playgrounds. Further, not only is salt heavily used in fast food, processed food, and artificial flavorings because it is a preservative but sodium in higher concentrations suppresses any bitterness in the flavor, which means the customer believes the food is tastier.[84] Hence the battle between health authorities and the salt and processed food industries.

Biohacking Your Sodium Genes

Sodium is an essential micronutrient that regulates blood pressure and blood volume, and the major adverse effect of excess sodium intake is elevated blood pressure, which in turn can lead to heart disease. However, some individuals do not experience as great an increase in blood pressure in response to excess sodium intake as others because the effect of sodium intake on blood pressure is influenced by variations in a gene called ACE.[85] The ACE gene directs the body to produce the angiotensin-converting enzyme, which is known to play a role in regulating the response of blood pressure to sodium intake. This is why some blood pressure medications are called ACE-inhibitors.

If you possess the GA or AA variant of the ACE gene, you are at a greater risk of experiencing elevated blood pressure, as confirmed by a study of elite athletes and people with hypertension.[86] For people with higher risk variants, it is even more important to follow the Dietary Reference Intake recommendations for adults to consume no more than 2,300 mg of sodium per day.[87] This equals about 5 g of salt per day, from all sources. However, if you frequently sweat heavily during exercise, causing sodium losses, your sodium requirements may be slightly higher. Foods that are high in sodium include canned soups, canned vegetables, potato chips, processed meats, soy sauce, ketchup, and processed cheeses. Aim to choose lower-sodium options of these high-sodium foods.

Food Sources High in Sodium[88]

Sources of Sodium	Amount (g)
Ramen noodles, chicken flavor, dry (1 package)	1760
Breakfast bagel with ham, egg, and cheese	1259
Chicken vegetable soup, chunky (250 mL)	1128
Ham, lean and regular, roasted (75 g)	1039
Pickle, cucumber, dill (65 g)	833

Tomato sauce, canned (125 mL)	678
Feta cheese (50 g)	558
Oatmeal, instant, apple-cinnamon (1 packet)	256
Potato chips, plain (1 small bag)	229
Bread, white, commercial (1 slice)	238

LAW 24

Babies given salt end up with a lifelong taste for salt. Sodium in salt increases blood pressure, and reducing salt reduces heart attacks and strokes. Salt is added as a preservative in processed foods and also helps suppress any bitter taste.

6

HACKS FOR HAPPINESS

We possess the power, to a great extent, of so exercising the will as to direct the thoughts upon objects calculated to yield happiness and improvement rather than their opposites.

—Samuel Smiles

Theodore Seward and the Story of the Don't Worry Movement

Theodore Seward was a musicologist and conductor of music in the late 1800s. In 1867, he conducted the Musical Pioneer in New York, and after a stint in London, he founded the American Tonic Sol-fa Association, which taught sight-singing using this system of music where the tones are called do, re, mi, fa, so, la, ti (Remember *The Sound of Music* film?[1]). In the late 1890s, Seward founded Don't Worry Clubs, a fad that lasted around thirty years. Rather than being merely about techniques taught about avoiding stress, Seward's clubs were essentially a Christian brotherhood sect, and he sold the Don't Worry doctrine as something founded by Jesus Christ.[2] It has long been known that worrying or feeling stressed can cause physical symptoms and Seventh Day Adventists' were particularly enthusiastic proponents of positive thinking.

Kelly McGonigal, psychologist at Stanford, has written a book titled, *The Upside of Stress: Why Stress Is Good for You, and How to Get Good at It.*[3] In the book, McGonigal talks about stress management and the power of considering it as a learning experiment. If someone can think that going through stress can make them better at handling it, it becomes easier and easier. And it turns out, the same is true for physical health—if you think stress is causing you ill health, it does; if you believe that stress cannot harm you, it doesn't!

A research group from Wisconsin studied the impact of stress on health. The starting point of the study was the beginning of the quarter in which they were interviewed for the 1998 National Health Interview Survey—a household questionnaire distributed by the department of statistics to over 150,000 people—that asked people about the amount of stress they were under, if they felt if affected their health, and if they had taken any steps to reduce stress. People were followed until 2006 when National Death Index mortality data were compared and matched with the interviewees.[4] What this study found was staggering: those who reported a lot of stress and felt that stress impacted their health a lot had a 43 percent increased risk of premature death, and those that reported similar stress but felt that stress could not harm their health did not have this same risk of dying prematurely. Approximately 33.7 percent of American adults self-reported that stress had an impact on their health.[5]

Stress evolved from our fight-or-flight response to danger. Stressful situations cause us to produce adrenaline (epinephrine), noradrenaline, and cortisol in that order. There is a distinction between acute (short-term) stress and chronic (longer-term) stress; the former may indeed be beneficial. After all, the stress response is an evolutionarily learned response to a particular memory, and many of the chemicals secreted help us cope with danger and adapt. Animal studies have shown that significant but brief stressful events cause stem cells in the brains to produce new brain cells and improve performance.[6] Essentially, short-term stress stimulates interleukins that boost our immunity and protect against illnesses; chronic stress, in contrast, lowers immunity and increases inflammation.[7]

A study done on over a hundred pregnant women showed that babies born to women who experienced mild to moderate stress during pregnancy had better developmental skills by the age of two when compared to those kids whose mothers had no stress. Therefore, mild to moderate stress in short bursts can be good for us as long as we think of it in that manner. And this is even transmitted to the baby. The children of women who regarded their pregnancy as a negative rather than a positive time showed slightly poorer emotional control and attention capacity.[8]

Therefore, when faced with stress, it is important to:

1. Think of the body response as normal given the situation you are in.
2. Be confident that you will not only get through this stress but be better for it.
3. Consider that stress is something everyone faces and is not unique to you.

Even if in the past you were someone who viewed stress as negative, by embracing stress as a positive factor, you can change your health for the better, and research shows that anyone can change their thinking around to this positive mindset. You don't need Seward's clubs after all.

Many years ago, I used to run an independent bookstore café, Baci Lounge. I remember seeing a book called *Living with a Black Dog*, an illustrated book referring to depression.[9] If one were to consider stress as a brown dog, the trick to dealing with it is in realizing that it may have a bark but no teeth to bite you. So, don't worry. Be happy.

Manifesting Happiness

> Before World War II, psychology had three missions:
> curing mental illness, making the lives of all people more
> fulfilling, and identifying and nurturing high talent. . . .
> Fifty years later, I want to remind our field . . . treatment
> is not just fixing what is broken, it is nurturing what is best
> within ourselves.
>
> —Martin Seligman

Being positive or optimistic can sometimes be aimless (i.e.,
"I am going to have a great day no matter what"). But studies
show that there are these thoughts that on their own cannot
lead to hope, and thereby personal progress. Hope, in my
view, is learned optimism with a plan. Success under this plan
involves three main components: goal, positivity, and agency
(the first two are self-explanatory; agency is when you have
control of your actions, in other words, have intentionality).

In medicine, we see the effects of positivity all the time. As
a skin doctor, I routinely perform skin biopsies. In 2004, a team
led by Marcel Ebrecht of Kings College, London, undertook a
study on men undergoing a punch biopsy, a common dermato-
logical procedure wherein a small cylindrical core of skin that
typically involves all the layers of skin is punched out using an
instrument. It turned out that your wound healing depended
on your thinking. The group was divided into slow and fast
healers based on their wound healing times. A simultaneous

assessment of mental thought processes was undertaken. The study showed that slow healers were significantly lower in optimism than fast healers. This was attributed to raised cortisol levels ,which we know happens during stressful situations.[10]

The Women's Health Initiative was a large-scale project in America involving thousands of women designed to study changes in and predictors of quality of life, chronic diseases, and death rates among women across America. From this cohort, an eight-year study looked at more than 97,000 women and analyzed the differences in health outcomes between those who were optimists and those who were pessimistic thinkers. The results were clear and dramatic. Over these eight years, optimists were not only less likely to develop coronary disease (reduced by 9 percent) but 30 percent less likely to die from heart disease.[11]

Over and over again, the evidence in medical studies is overwhelming. A study from Wageningen University in Holland of nine hundred women found that optimists were less likely to die in the next ten years from any cause.[12]

So, how does one cultivate positive thinking and hopeful optimism for greater success? Following the steps I have outlined next is a good guide. This is something I use when mentoring medical colleagues, students, and even school children.

I use VIGOUR as a useful mnemonic to help them remember these steps. (Please excuse the UK spelling. After all, I was born in England!)

V: Visualize success—Think of your goals and how you are going to achieve them—the plan and your actions.

I: Increase self-awareness—Known techniques for developing self-awareness are meditation and practiced breathing. Even keeping a daily journal can help.

G: Gratitude—Simple practiced gratitude like complimenting yourself and others; being grateful for people in your life and letting them know that. In a business, being grateful to and for your customers.

O: Optimism orbit—Hang out or spend time with positive people and avoid those who drag you down with their negativity.

U: Understanding—Essentially, understanding negativity is reframing your thinking. For example, if you are anxious about an exam, you can change your thinking to "I am not the only one. It is normal to feel this way. What's the worst that can happen? Eventually things are going to work out fine."

R: Reinforcement—This is where using external resources helps. Watching a comedy, buying something for yourself, or receiving gifts, etc.

Such practiced positivity helps not only your healthspan but also your lifespan.

Biohacking Your Negative Genes for Happiness

I have discussed DNA methylation from the context of aging previously. In this chapter, we have been discussing the differences between positive and negative thinkers. What we now know is there are genetic variations between groups and our thinking alters our genes. DNA methylation is known to be involved in the regulation of stress-related gene expression, and a particular enzyme, DNMT3A, is involved in how your brain mediates and regulates such emotional processes.

A research study—even if a small observational one—looked at genetic variations between positive and negative thinkers and concluded that consistent patterns were observed for only one genetic variation (rs11683424 in the DNMT3A gene). People who carried the T-allele (CT or TT variant of the gene) of rs11683424 can buffer the impact of daily stressful events on negative affect.[13] Buffering in mental health refers to positivity or processes that can ward of ill health.

We therefore know that some people are genetically more inclined to be positive thinkers. But we also know that practising positivity using the framework I explained earlier can help you alter your genes, and such epigenetics can lead to happiness and hopefulness no matter what your gene type. Ultimately, science suggests that we can improve our health and control our life favorably as we are living it. It takes some effort, but there is something enjoyable that comes with the eudurance of this work: a better life.

LAW 25

The way you think—positive or negative—can affect not only your health but also your lifespan. There are methods in which you can learn optimistic and hopeful thinking, irrespective of your gene type.

Appendix

The Gene-Testing Program for Better Health and Skin

As a skin MD and scientist, I have often said to my patients, "One cannot have good health and bad skin." And also: "Genes are our blueprint, but not our destiny." Genes are essentially protein makers, and if we eat and do the right things, we make helpful proteins; if we eat stuff that is not good for us, we end up with bad proteins and poor health.

But how do we know what we should eat? This isn't intuitive. Let's take a simple example: coffee. A cup of coffee after midday keeps me up at night, and I assumed I had dodgy caffeine genes. It turns out my caffeine genes are fine, and coffee is good for me. But until I tested my own genes, I had no idea.

In a mission to biohack genes for better health for myself and my patients, I have developed a comprehensive gene-testing program that is all about wellness: what it tells you is all about eating and exercising specifically for your gene type. The latest version of our gene-testing program is now ready.

Soon, you will also be able to order supplements tailored specifically for you. Science suggests that taking supplements without a specific deficiency or understanding your specific risk factors may be meaningless.

The Dermatogenomix® test is about analyzing your genetic code to determine what is best for you and to provide individual recommendations for better skin and health and to help you understand your food intolerances, improve your fitness performance, and lower your injury risk. You can become a super-ager!

In my lab, we do not test for any illnesses, so no worries regarding your insurance premiums or future illnesses. This is all about prevention—eating and exercising for your gene type—and your own personal evolution into a new, healthier you! For further information, or if you would like to order your gene test, visit www.biohackingyourgenes.com.

Tailored Supplements for Your Gene Type

I have often joked that taking too many supplements only creates expensive urine, and our human body is pretty good at rejecting what it does not need. As I have noted repeatedly in this book, I'm all about healthspan, not lifespan for the sake of it.

In 2017, we began our gene-testing for wellness programs out of my lab alongside my previous book, *The Genetics of Health*. From data analyzed from thousands of our clients all across the globe, I have found that, broadly, people come under three categories (i.e., with a higher risk of the following deficiencies), and therefore, my research lab has created a range of tailored supplements, with precise formulations, gleaned from these seven years of research.

Groups at Risk of Deficiencies and Recommended Supplements

Supplement Group	Main Ingredients	Main Benefits
Vitamin D Group	Vitamin D, Lutein, Xeazanthin, Coenzyme Q10	Musculoskeletal, eye health, and energy systems
Vitamin B Group	Folate, B12, Magnesium, and Zinc	Blood cell and heart health, sleep, and immune function
Vitamin C Group	Vitamin C, Hyaluronic acid, and Glucosamine	Skin and bone health, collagen production

If you undertake the Dermatogenomix® gene-testing program, your results will dictate what type of supplements are best for you.

Notes

Introduction

1. Frederick Golden, "Shaping Life in the Lab," *Time*, March 9, 1981, https://time.com/archive/6854882/shaping-life-in-the-lab/.

Chapter 1

1. Darren Aronofsky and Ari Handel, "Memory," *Limitless with Chris Hemsworth*, episode 5, directed by Kit Lynch Robinson and Jens Schollmoller, featuring Chris Hemsworth, Peter Attia, and Otis Hope Carey, aired November 16, 2022, on Disney+ and Apple TV.

2. "Study Finds Differences in APOE ε4 Expression Based on Genetic Ancestry," National Institute on Aging, July 1, 2021, https://www.nia.nih.gov/news/study-finds-differences-apoe -e4-expression-based-genetic-ancestry.

3. Anthony J. Griswold et al., "Increased APOE ε4 Expression Is Associated with the Difference in Alzheimer's Disease Risk from Diverse Ancestral Backgrounds," *Alzheimer's & Dementia* 17, no. 7 (July 2021): 1179–88, https://doi.org/10.1002/alz.12287.

4. Akinori Miyashita et al., "Genetics of Alzheimer's Disease: An East Asian Perspective," *Journal of Human Genetics* 68 (June 1, 2022): 115–24, https://doi.org/10.1038/s10038-022-01050-z.

5. David Mouriquand, "Chris Hemsworth Taking Break from Acting After Revealing Alzheimer's Risk," *Euronews*, November 20, 2022, https://www.euronews.com/culture/2022/11/20 /chris-hemsworth-taking-break-from-acting-after-revealing-alzheimers-risk.

6. Glenn Campbell, "Glen Campbell in 2022: 'I'm a Cheap High'," interview by Larry King, CNN, April 7, 2002, https:// www.celebstoner.com/news/celebstoner-news/2017/08/09 /glen-campbell-on-tobacco-cocaine-alcohol/.

7. Ronald Petersen, quoted in Damian Garde, "Fans 'Didn't Care if He Messed Up': Glen Campbell's Doctor Discusses His Struggle with Alzheimer's," *Stat News*, August 9, 2017, https://www .statnews.com/2017/08/09/glen-campbell-alzheimers/.

8. Ronald Petersen, quoted in Garde, "Fans 'Didn't Care if He Messed Up'."

9. George S. Bloom, "Amyloid-β and Tau: The Trigger and Bullet in Alzheimer Disease Pathogenesis," *JAMA Neurology* 71, no. 4 (April 2014): 505, https://doi.org/10.1001/jamaneurol.2013.5847.

10. Sylvain Lesné et al., "A Specific Amyloid-β Protein Assembly in the Brain Impairs Memory," *Nature* 440 (March 16, 2006): 352–57, https://doi.org/10.1038/nature04533.

11. Charles Piller, "Blots on a Field?" *Science*, July 21, 2022, https://www.science.org/content/article/potential-fabrication -research-images-threatens-key-theory-alzheimers-disease.

12. Piller, "Blots on a Field?"

13. Piller, "Blots on a Field?"

14. Piller, "Blots on a Field?"

15. Cláudio Gouveia Roque et al., "CREB3L2-ATF4 Hetero-dimerization Defines a Transcriptional Hub of Alzheimer's

Disease Gene Expression Linked to Neuropathology," *Science Advance* 9, no. 9 (March 3, 2023), https://www.science.org /doi/10.1126/sciadv.add2671.

16. Martha Clare Morris et al., "MIND Diet Associated with Reduced Incidence of Alzheimer's Disease," *Alzheimer's & Dementia: The Journal of the Alzheimer's Association* 11, no. 9 (2015): 1010, https://doi.org/10.1016/j.jalz.2014.11.009.

17. Whitney Wharton et al., "A Pilot Randomized Clinical Trial of Adapted Tango to Improve Cognition and Psychosocial Function in African American Women with Family History of Alzheimer's Disease (ACT Trial)," *Cerebral Circulation— Cognition and Behavior* 2 (2021): 1–9, https://doi.org/10.1016/j .cccb.2021.100018.

18. Emma Swanwick and Martyn Matthews, "Energy Systems: A New Look at Aerobic Metabolism in Stressful Exercise," *MOJ Sports Medicine* 2, no. 1 (January 19, 2018): 15, fig. 1, https://doi .org/10.15406/mojsm.2018.02.00039.

19. Dr. Neubauer Table Tennis, accessed December 21, 2023, https:// www.drneubauer.com/.

20. Scott Culpin, "Effects of Long-Term Participation in Tennis on Cognitive Function in Elderly Individuals" (Master's Thesis, Edith Cowan University, 2018), https://ro.ecu.edu.au /theses/2097/.

21. Jon Wertheim, "Novak Djokovic Says Hungry, Young Tennis Players 'Awaken a Beast' in Him," *60 Minutes*, CBS News, December 10, 2023, https://www.cbsnews.com/news/novak -djokovic-hungry-young-tennis-players-awaken-beast-60 -minutes-transcript/.

22. Martha Clare Morris et al., "MIND Diet Slows Cognitive Decline with Aging," *Alzheimer's & Dementia* 11, no. 9 (September 2015): 1015, https://doi.org/10.1016/j.jalz.2015.04.011.

23. Martha Clare Morris et al., "Nutrients and Bioactives in Green Leafy Vegetables and Cognitive Decline," *Neurology* 90, no. 3 (January 16, 2018): e214, https://doi.org/10.1212/WNL.0000000000004815.

24. Morris et al., "MIND Diet Slows Cognitive Decline with Aging," e214.

25. "Martha Clare Morris Details Her MIND Diet for Healthy Brain Aging at 2017 Fall Lecture," Alzheimer's Disease Research Center, University of Wisconsin Madison, November 1, 2017, https://www.adrc.wisc.edu/news/martha-clare-morris-details-her-mind-diet-healthy-brain-aging-2017-fall-lecture.

26. Walter Willett et al, "Food in the Anthropocene: The EAT–Lancet Commission on Healthy Diets from Sustainable Food Systems," *The Lancet* 393, no. 10170 (January 16, 2019): 447–92, https://doi.org/10.1016/s0140-6736(18)31788-4.

27. Huifeng Zhang, Janet Cade, and Laura Hadie, "Consumption of Red Meat Is Negatively Associated with Cognitive Function: A Cross-Sectional Analysis of UK Biobank," *Current Developments in Nutrition* 4, no. 2 (June 2020): 1510, https://doi.org/10.1093/cdn/nzaa061_138.

28. Carla Harris et al., "Prospective Associations of Meat Consumption During Childhood with Measures of Body Composition During Adolescence: Results from the GINIplus and LISAplus Birth Cohorts," *Nutrition Journal* 15, no. 1 (December 2016): 9, https://doi.org/10.1186/s12937-016-0222-5.

29. C.P. Chong et al., "Habitual Sugar Intake and Cognitive Impairment among Multi-Ethnic Malaysian Older Adults," *Clinical Interventions in Aging* 14 (July 22, 2019): 1340, https://doi.org/10.2147/CIA.S211534.

30. Xingwang Ye et al., "Habitual Sugar Intake and Cognitive Function among Middle-Aged and Older Puerto Ricans Without

Diabetes," *British Journal of Nutrition* 106, no. 9 (November 14, 2011): 1431, https://doi.org/10.1017/S0007114511001760.

31. Matthew P. Pase et al., "Sugar- and Artificially Sweetened Beverages and the Risks of Incident Stroke and Dementia," *Stroke* 48, no. 5 (May 2017): 1144, https://doi.org/10.1161/strokeaha.116.016027.

32. Eleanor Wood et al., "Wild Blueberry (Poly)phenols Can Improve Vascular Function and Cognitive Performance in Healthy Older Individuals: A Double-Blind Randomized Controlled Trial," *The American Journal of Clinical Nutrition* 117, no. 6 (June 2023): 1306–19, https://doi.org/10.1016/j.ajcnut.2023.03.017.

33. Katie L. Barfoot et al., "The Effects of Acute Wild Blueberry Supplementation on the Cognition of 7–10-Year-Old Schoolchildren," *European Journal of Nutrition* 58 (October 16, 2019): 2911, https://doi.org/10.1007/s00394-018-1843-6.

34. Xin Xu et al., "Tofu Intake Is Associated with Poor Cognitive Performance among Community-Dwelling Elderly in China," *Journal of Alzheimer's Disease* 43, no. 2 (November 21, 2014): 669, https://doi.org/10.3233/jad-141593.

35. Carlotta Giromini and D. Ian Givens, "Benefits and Risks Associated with Meat Consumption during Key Life Processes and in Relation to the Risk of Chronic Diseases," *Foods* 11, no. 14 (January 1, 2022): 2063, https://doi.org/10.3390/foods11142063.

36. Panrapee Suttiwan et al., "Effectiveness of Essence of Chicken on Cognitive Function Improvement: A Randomized Controlled Clinical Trial," *Nutrients* 10, no. 7 (June 29, 2018): 845, https://doi.org/10.3390/nu10070845.

37. Richard P. Evershed et al., "Dairying, Diseases and the Evolution of Lactase Persistence in Europe," *Nature* 608, no. 7922 (August 1, 2022): 336, https://doi.org/10.1038/s41586-022-05010-7; Sharad P. Paul, MD, *The Genetics of Health* (Portland, OR: Beyond Words, 2017), 202–3.

38. Yair Field et al., "Detection of Human Adaptation during the Past 2000 Years," *Science* 354, no. 6313 (November 11, 2016): 763, https://doi.org/10.1126/science.aag0776.

39. Nick Patterson et al., "Large-Scale Migration into Britain during the Middle to Late Bronze Age," *Nature* 601 (January 27, 2022): 588, https://doi.org/10.1038/s41586-021-04287-4.

40. Shruti V. Baadkar, Manjari S. Mukherjee, and Smita S. Lele, "Study on Influence of Age, Gender and Genetic Variants on Lactose Intolerance and Its Impact on Milk Intake in Adult Asian Indians," *Annals of Human Biology* 41, no. 6 (April 15, 2014): 548, https://doi.org/10.3109/03014460.2014.902992; P. H. Kwon, Marvin H. Rorick, and Nevin S. Scrimshaw, "Comparative Tolerance of Adolescents of Differing Ethnic Backgrounds to Lactose-Containing and Lactose-Free Dairy Drinks. II. Improvement of a Double-Blind Test," *The American Journal of Clinical Nutrition* 33, no. 1 (January 1, 1980): 22, https://doi.org/10.1093/ajcn/33.1.22.

41. Natalia Petruski-Ivleva et al., "Milk Intake at Midlife and Cognitive Decline Over 20 Years. The Atherosclerosis Risk in Communities (ARIC) Study," *Nutrients* 9, no. 10 (October 17, 2017): 1134, https://doi.org/10.3390/nu9101134.

42. A. Rahman et al., "Dietary Factors and Cognitive Impairment in Community-Dwelling Elderly," *Journal of Nutrition, Health, and Aging* 11, no. 1 (January–February 2007): 49, https://pubmed.ncbi.nlm.nih.gov/17315080/.

43. Yuni Choi et al., "Vegetable Intake, but Not Fruit Intake, Is Associated with a Reduction in the Risk of Cancer Incidence and Mortality in Middle-Aged Korean Men," *The Journal of Nutrition* 145, no. 6 (June 2015): 1249, https://doi.org/10.3945/jn.114.209437.

44. Julia L. Bienias et al., "Design of the Chicago Health and Aging Project (CHAP)," *Journal of Alzheimer's Disease* 5, no. 5 (November 17, 2003): 349–55, https://doi.org/10.3233/jad-2003-5501.

45. Martha Clare Morris et al., "Nutrients and Bioactives in Green Leafy Vegetables and Cognitive Decline," e214.

46. Carmen Freire et al., "Hair Mercury Levels, Fish Consumption, and Cognitive Development in Preschool Children from Granada, Spain," *Environmental Research* 110, no. 1 (January 2010): 96, https://doi.org/10.1016/j.envres.2009.10.005.

47. A. Lehner et al., "Fish Consumption Is Associated with School Performance in Children in a Non-Linear Way: Results from the German Cohort Study Kiggs," *Evolution, Medicine, and Public Health* 2020, no. 1 (December 23, 2019): 2, https://doi.org/10.1093/emph/eoz038.

48. A. D. Dangour et al., "Fish Consumption and Cognitive Function among Older People in the UK: Baseline Data from the OPAL Study," *The Journal of Nutrition, Health and Aging* 13 (May 10, 2009): 198, https://doi.org/10.1007/s12603-009-0057-2.

49. Yuya Akagi et al., "Alcohol Drinking Patterns Have a Positive Association with Cognitive Function among Older People: A Cross-Sectional Study," *BMC Geriatrics* 22, (February 28, 2022): 158, https://doi.org/10.1186/s12877-022-02852-8.

50. Maribel Lucerón-Lucas-Torres et al., "Association Between Wine Consumption and Cognitive Decline in Older People: A Systematic Review and Meta-Analysis of Longitudinal Studies," *Frontiers in Nutrition* 9, (May 12, 2022): 863059, https://doi.org/10.3389/fnut.2022.863059.

51. L. Lee et al., "Relationships Between Dietary Intake and Cognitive Function Level in Korean Elderly People," *Public Health* 115, no. 2 (March 2001): 133, https://doi.org/10.1038/sj.ph.1900729.

52. Peter Pribis et al., "Effects of Walnut Consumption on Cognitive Performance in Young Adults," *British Journal of Nutrition* 107, no. 9 (May 14, 2012): 1393, https://doi.org/10.1017/S0007114511004302.

53. Jelena Mustra Rakic et al., "Effects of Daily Almond Consumption for Six Months on Cognitive Measures in Healthy Middle-Aged to Older Adults: A Randomized Control Trial," *Nutritional Neuroscience* 25, no. 7 (January 15, 2021): 1466, https://doi.org/10.1080/1028415x.2020.1868805.

54. Ming Li and Z. Shi, "A Prospective Association of Nut Consumption with Cognitive Function in Chinese Adults Aged 55+_China Health and Nutrition Survey," *The Journal of Nutrition, Health & Aging* 23, no. 2 (February 2019): 211, https://doi.org/10.1007/s12603-018-1122-5.

55. Holly C. Miller et al., "A Mind Cleared by Walnut Oil: The Effects of Polyunsaturated and Saturated Fat on Extinction Learning," *Appetite* 126 (July 1, 2018): 147, https://doi.org/10.1016/j.appet.2018.04.004.

56. Lei An et al., "Walnut Diets Up-Regulate the Decreased Hippocampal Neurogenesis and Age-Related Cognitive Dysfunction in D-Galactose Induced Aged Rats," *Food & Function* 9, no. 9 (January 1, 2018): 4755, https://doi.org/10.1039/c8fo00702k.

57. Abha Chauhan and Ved Chauhan, "Beneficial Effects of Walnuts on Cognition and Brain Health," *Nutrients* 12, no. 2 (February 20, 2020): 550, https://doi.org/10.3390/nu12020550.

58. Antonia Chiou and Nick Kalogeropoulos, "Virgin Olive Oil as Frying Oil," *Comprehensive Reviews in Food Science and Food Safety* 16, no. 4 (July 2017): 632, https://doi.org/10.1111/1541-4337.12268.

59. Elisa Mazza et al., "Effect of the Replacement of Dietary Vegetable Oils with a Low Dose of Extra Virgin Olive Oil in the Mediterranean Diet on Cognitive Functions in the Elderly," *Journal of*

Translational Medicine 16, no. 1 (January 19, 2018): 10, https://doi.org/10.1186/s12967-018-1386-x.

Chapter 2

1. "David Rudisha," Athletes, World Athletics, accessed October 26, 2023, https://worldathletics.org/athletes/kenya/david-rudisha-14209691.
2. Paul, "The Pigment Genes: The Myth of Race" in *The Genetics of Health*, 145–78.
3. Jason Henderson, "Great Moments—Coe vs Ovett in 1980," *Athletics Weekly*, December 13, 2020, https://athleticsweekly.com/featured/great-moments-coe-vs-ovett-in-1980-1039938385/.
4. Matt Long, "How They Trained—Learning from the Greats," *Athletics Weekly*, January 23, 2021, https://athleticsweekly.com/performance/learning-from-the-greats-1039939767/.
5. Gareth N. Sandford et al., "Tactical Behaviors in Men's 800-m Olympic and World-Championship Medalists: A Changing of the Guard," *International Journal of Sports Physiology and Performance* 13, no. 2 (February 1, 2018): 246–49, https://doi.org/10.1123/ijspp.2016-0780.
6. Arturo Casado et al., "Pacing Profiles and Tactical Behaviors of Elite Runners," *Journal of Sport and Health Science* 10, no. 5 (September 2021): 537–49, https://doi.org/10.1016/j.jshs.2020.06.011.
7. *Man on a Mission: Born to Run*, directed by Maurice Sweeney, produced by Jamie D'Alton and Anne McLoughlin, presented by Eamonn Coghlan, featuring Colm O'Connell, 52 min., aired July 2012 on BBC Four, https://www.motive.ie/portfolio-posts/man-on-a-mission-born-to-run/.

8. Martine F. Luxwolda et al., "Traditionally Living Populations in East Africa Have a Mean Serum 25-Hydroxyvitamin D Concentration of 115 nmol/l," *British Journal of Nutrition* 108, no. 9 (November 14, 2012): 1557, https://doi.org/10.1017/S0007114511007161.

9. Nikolaos E. Koundourakis et al., "Vitamin D and Exercise Performance in Professional Soccer Players," *PLOS ONE* 9, no. 7 (July 3, 2014): e101659, https://doi.org/10.1371/journal.pone.0101659.

10. Julias Maina Mathara et al., "Functional Characteristics of Lactobacillus spp. From Traditional Maasai Fermented Milk Products in Kenya," *International Journal of Food Microbiology* 126, no. 1–2 (August 15, 2008): 62, https://doi.org/10.1016/j.ijfoodmicro.2008.04.027.

11. Katarzyna Przewłócka et al., "Effects of Probiotics and Vitamin D3 Supplementation on Sports Performance Markers in Male Mixed Martial Arts Athletes: A Randomized Trial," *Sports Medicine* 9, no. 1 (May 16, 2023): 31, https://doi.org/10.1186/s40798-023-00576-6.

12. Kimberly Y. Z. Forrest and Wendy L. Stuhldreher, "Prevalence and Correlates of Vitamin D Deficiency in US Adults," *Nutrition Research* 31, no. 1 (January 2011): 48, https://doi.org/10.1016/j.nutres.2010.12.001.

13. Alaa Abdeldaiem, "Olympic Champion David Rudisha Survives Head-On Car Accident in Kenya," *Sports Illustrated*, August 26, 2019, https://www.si.com/olympics/2019/08/26/david-rudisha-survives-car-accident-kenya.

14. Simon Turnbull, "Remembering Rudisha's 'Gun to Tape' World Record Run in London," World Athletics Heritage, Museum of World Athletics, August 9, 2022, https://worldathletics.org/heritage/news/david-rudisha-kenya-world-800m-record-london-2012-olympic-games.

15. Martina Barnevik-Olsson, Christopher Gillberg, and Elisabeth Fernell, "Prevalence of Autism in Children Born to Somali Parents Living in Sweden: A Brief Report," *Developmental Medicine & Child Neurology* 50, no. 8 (August 2008): 598, https://doi .org/10.1111/j.1469-8749.2008.03036.x.

16. Irva Hertz-Picciotto and Lora Delwiche, "The Rise in Autism and the Role of Age at Diagnosis," *Epidemiology* 20, no. 1 (January 2009): 84, https://doi.org/10.1097/ede.0b013e3181902d15.

17. Simon Baron-Cohen et al., "Foetal Oestrogens and Autism," *Molecular Psychiatry* 25 (July 29, 2019): 2970–78, https://doi .org/10.1038/s41380-019-0454-9.

18. Yanan Luo et al., "Urbanicity and Autism of Children in China," *Psychiatry Research* 286, no. 7 (February 2020): 112867, https:// doi.org/10.1016/j.psychres.2020.112867.

19. C. L. Muller, A. M. J. Anacker, and J. Veenstra-VanderWeele, "The Serotonin System in Autism Spectrum Disorder: From Biomarker to Animal Models," *Neuroscience* 321 (May 2016): 24–41, https://doi.org/10.1016/j.neuroscience.2015.11.010.

20. Muller et al., "The Serotonin System in Autism Spectrum Disorder."

21. Rhonda P. Patrick and Bruce N. Ames, "Vitamin D Hormone Regulates Serotonin Synthesis. Part 1: Relevance for Autism," *Federation of American Societies for Experimental Biology (FASEB) Journal* 28, no. 6 (June 2014): 2398–413, https://doi .org/10.1096/fj.13-246546.

22. Michael Waldman et al., "Autism Prevalence and Precipitation Rates in California, Oregon, and Washington Counties," *Archives of Pediatric and Adolescent Medicine* 162, no. 11 (November 3, 2008): 1026, https://doi.org/10.1001 /archpedi.162.11.1026.

23. Baris Karsli, "Comparative Analysis of the Fatty Acid Composition of Commercially Available Fish Oil Supplements in

Turkey: Public Health Risks and Benefits," *Journal of Food Composition and Analysis* 103 (July 2021): 104105, https://doi.org/10.1016/j.jfca.2021.104105.

24. Ran Zhang and Declan P Naughton, "Vitamin D in Health and Disease: Current Perspectives," *Nutrition Journal* 9, no. 65 (December 2010): 1, https://doi.org/10.1186/1475-2891-9-65.

25. A. P. Simopoulos, "The Importance of the Ratio of Omega-6/Omega-3 Essential Fatty Acids," *Biomedicine & Pharmacotherapy* 56, no. 8 (October 2002): 365, https://doi.org/10.1016/s0753-3322(02)00253-6.

26. Joseph V. Ferraro et al., "Earliest Archaeological Evidence of Persistent Hominin Carnivory," *PLOS ONE* 8, no. 4 (April 25, 2013): e62174, https://doi.org/10.1371/journal.pone.0062174.

27. Michael Weiser, Christopher Butt, and M. Mohajeri, "Docosahexaenoic Acid and Cognition throughout the Lifespan," *Nutrients* 8, no. 2 (February 17, 2016): 99, https://doi.org/10.3390/nu8020099.

28. Narinder Kaur, Vishal Chugh, and Anil K. Gupta, "Essential Fatty Acids as Functional Components of Foods—A Review," *Journal of Food Science and Technology* 51, no. 10 (March 21, 2012): 2290, https://doi.org/10.1007/s13197-012-0677-0.

29. Kaur, Chugh, and Gupta, "Essential Fatty Acids as Functional Components of Foods," 2289.

30. Dawn M. Richard, Michael A. Dawes et al., "L-Tryptophan: Basic Metabolic Functions, Behavioral Research and Therapeutic Indications," *International Journal of Tryptophan Research* 2 (March 23, 2009): 46, table 1, https://doi.org/10.4137/IJTR.S2129.

31. Hajar Mazahery et al., "A Randomised Controlled Trial of Vitamin D and Omega-3 Long Chain Polyunsaturated Fatty Acids in the Treatment of Irritability and Hyperactivity among Children with Autism Spectrum Disorder," *The Journal of Steroid*

Biochemistry and Molecular Biology 187 (March 2019): 9, https://doi.org/10.1016/j.jsbmb.2018.10.017.

32. Yunru Huang et al., "Maternal Polyunsaturated Fatty Acids and Risk for Autism Spectrum Disorder in the *MARBLES* High-Risk Study," *Autism* 24, no. 5 (July 2020): 1191, https://doi.org/10.1177/1362361319877792.

33. Huang et al., "Maternal Polyunsaturated Fatty Acids and Risk for Autism Spectrum Disorder," 1196.

34. Huang et al., "Maternal Polyunsaturated Fatty Acids and Risk for Autism Spectrum Disorder," 1196.

35. Herodotus, "Book III: Thalia," in A *New and Literal Version from the Text of Baehr: With a Geographical and General Index By Henry Cary* (New York: Harper & Brothers, Publishers, 1859), 170–171, https://archive.org/details/herodotusnewlite00hero/page/174/mode/2up.

36. Herodotus, "Book III: Thalia," 174.

37. Herodotus, "Book III: Thalia," 174.

38. E. V. Wilcox, "Effect of Sunlight on Bone as Reported by Herodotus in 450 B. C.," *Journal of the American Medical Association* 112, no. 19 (May 13, 1939): 1987, https://doi.org/10.1001/jama.1939.02800190101027.

39. Eugene J. Kucharz, MD, PhD, Marc A. Shampo, PhdD, and Robert A. Kyle, MD, "Casimir Funk—Polish-Born American Biochemist," *Mayo Clinic Proceedings* 69, no. 7 (July 1994): 656, https://doi.org/10.1016/S0025-6196(12)61343-3. In the early 1900s, chemists thought these substances were all chemically amines, which we know now they are not.

40. In medicine, endocrine relates to organs or glands where hormones or chemicals are secreted directly into the bloodstream. Autocrine means a cell secreting a chemical substance that binds to the receptors on the same cell, causing functional changes in the

cell. Paracrine is when the target cell is located close to the signal-releasing cell.

41. Wedad Z. Mostafa and Rehab A. Hegazy, "Vitamin D and the Skin: Focus on a Complex Relationship: A Review," *Journal of Advanced Research* 6, no. 6 (November 2015): 793, https://doi.org/10.1016/j.jare.2014.01.011.

42. Sharad P. Paul, *Skin: A Biography* (Gurugram, Haryana: Harper-Collins Publishers India, 2013), 11.

43. Irina Terenetskaya et al., "Action Spectrum for the Production of Previtamin D3 in Human Skin," International Commission on Illumination (January 2006): 1–12, https://www.researchgate.net/publication/258069304_Action_Spectrum_for_the_Production_of_Pre-Vitamin_D_in_Human_Skin; T. C. B. Stamp, J. G. Haddad, and C. A. Twigg, "Comparison of Oral 25-Hydroxycholecalciferol, Vitamin D, and Ultraviolet Light as Determinants of Circulating 25-Hydroxyvitamin D," *The Lancet* 309, no. 8026 (June 1977): 1341, https://doi.org/10.1016/s0140-6736(77)92553-3.

44. David R. Fraser, "Physiological Significance of Vitamin D Produced in Skin Compared with Oral Vitamin D," *Journal of Nutritional Science* 11 (January 18, 2022): 3, table 2, https://doi.org/10.1017/jns.2022.11.

45. Eliot T. Obi-Tabot et al., "A Human Skin Equivalent Model That Mimics the Photoproduction of Vitamin D3 in Human Skin," *In Vitro Cellular & Developmental Biology—Animal* 36, no. 3 (March 2000): 201, https://doi.org/10.1290/1071-2690(2000)036%3C0201:ahsemt%3E2.0.co;2.

46. Paul Urbain and Jette Jakobsen, "Dose–Response Effect of Sunlight on Vitamin D2 Production in Agaricus Bisporus Mushrooms," *Journal of Agricultural and Food Chemistry* 63, no. 37 (September 11, 2015): 8156, https://doi.org/10.1021/acs.jafc.5b02945.

47. Rakesh Balachandar et al.,"Relative Efficacy of Vitamin D2 and Vitamin D3 in Improving Vitamin D Status: Systematic Review and Meta-Analysis," *Nutrients* 13, no. 10 (September 23, 2021): 3328, https://doi.org/10.3390/nu13103328.

48. Fraser, "Physiological Significance of Vitamin D Produced in Skin Compared with Oral Vitamin D," 2, table 1.

49. Vu Tran et al., "Vitamin D and Sun Exposure: A Community Survey in Australia," *Current Oncology* 30, no. 2 (February 2023): 2465, https://doi.org/10.3390/curroncol30020188.

50. Andrea Quadri et al., "Seasonal Variation of Vitamin D Levels in Swiss Athletes," *Swiss Sports & Exercise Medicine* 64, no. 1 (2016): 24, https://doi.org/10.34045/ssem/2016/2.

51. Josephine Marcotty, "Sunday: Doctor Preaches Wonder Cure: Vitamin D," *Star Tribune*, September 22, 2008, https://www.startribune.com/sunday-minnesota-doctor-preaches-wonder-cure-vitamin-d/28701254/.

52. "The Myth of Race | Sharad Paul | TEDxAuckland," TEDx Talks, video, Auckland, New Zealand, 18:10, July 14, 2016, https://www.youtube.com/watch?v=8v0ykTrTQEc.

53. Paul, *The Genetics of Health*, 158–59.

54. Ristya Widi Endah Yani et al., "Analysis of Calcium Levels in Groundwater and Dental Caries in the Coastal Population of an Archipelago Country," *Open Access Macedonian Journal of Medical Sciences* 7, no. 1 (January 13, 2019): 135, https://doi.org/10.3889/oamjms.2019.013.

55. EFSA Panel on Dietetic Products, Nutrition and Allergies (NDA), "Scientific Opinion on Dietary Reference Values for Phosphorus," *EFSA Journal* 13, no. 7 (July 2015): 1–2, https://doi.org/10.2903/j.efsa.2015.4185.

56. Kamyar Kalantar-Zadeh et al., "Understanding Sources of Dietary Phosphorus in the Treatment of Patients with Chronic Kidney Disease," *Clinical Journal of the American Society of Nephrology*

5, no. 3 (January 21, 2010): 519, https://doi.org/10.2215/cjn.06080809.

57. Erik-Jan Lock et al., "The Vitamin D Receptor and Its Ligand 1α,25-Dihydroxyvitamin D3 in Atlantic Salmon (Salmo Salar)," *Journal of Endocrinology* 193, no. 3 (June 1, 2007): 459, https://doi.org/10.1677/joe-06-0198.

58. Swati, "The Indian 'RxEvolutionary' Approach to Modern Healthcare," *The Sunday Guardian Live*, June 3, 2017, https://sundayguardianlive.com/lifestyle/9626-indian-rxevolutionary-approach-modern-healthcare.

59. Anastassios G. Pittas et al., "The Role of Vitamin D and Calcium in Type 2 Diabetes. A Systematic Review and Meta-Analysis," *The Journal of Clinical Endocrinology & Metabolism* 92, no. 6 (June 2007): 2017–29, https://doi.org/10.1210/jc.2007-0298.

60. Mahmoud Barbarawi et al., "Vitamin D Supplementation and Cardiovascular Disease Risks in More than 83 000 Individuals in 21 Randomized Clinical Trials," *JAMA Cardiology* 4, no. 8 (June 19, 2019): 765–76, https://doi.org/10.1001/jamacardio.2019.1870.

61. "Skin Cancer Facts & Statistics," National Council on Skin Cancer Prevention," accessed December 21, 2023, https://skincancerprevention.org/learning/melanoma-facts-statistics/.

62. Maria N. Ombra et al., "Vitamin D Status and Risk for Malignant Cutaneous Melanoma: Recent Advances," *European Journal of Cancer Prevention* 26, no. 6 (November 2017): 532, https://doi.org/10.1097/cej.0000000000000334.

63. Emilia Kanasuo et al., "Regular Use of Vitamin D Supplement Is Associated with Fewer Melanoma Cases Compared to Non-Use: A Cross-Sectional Study in 498 Adult Subjects at Risk of Skin Cancers," *Melanoma Research* 33, no. 2 (December 28, 2022): 126, https://doi.org/10.1097/CMR.0000000000000870.

64. Zengrong Wu, Deliang Liu, and Feihong Deng, "The Role of Vitamin D in Immune System and Inflammatory Bowel Disease," *Journal of Inflammation Research* 2022, no. 15 (May 2022): 3167–85, https://doi.org/10.2147/jir.s363840.

65. Wu et al., "The Role of Vitamin D in Immune System and Inflammatory Bowel Disease," 3177.

66. Jill Hahn et al., "Vitamin D and Marine Omega 3 Fatty Acid Supplementation and Incident Autoimmune Disease: VITAL Randomized Controlled Trial," *British Medical Journal* 2022, no. 376 (January 26, 2022): e066452, https://doi.org/10.1136/bmj-2021-066452.

67. Hahn, et al. "Vitamin D and Marine Omega 3 Fatty Acid Supplementation and Incident Autoimmune Disease: VITAL Randomized Controlled Trial," 1.

68. Nipith Charoenngam, "Vitamin D and Rheumatic Diseases: A Review of Clinical Evidence," *International Journal of Molecular Sciences* 22, no. 19 (October 1, 2021): 10659, https://doi.org/10.3390/ijms221910659.

69. Linlin Yang et al., "Therapeutic Effect of Vitamin D Supplementation in a Pilot Study of Crohn's Patients," *Clinical and Translational Gastroenterology* 4, no. 4 (April 2013): e33, https://doi.org/10.1038/ctg.2013.1.

70. Mislav Radić et al., "Vitamin D and Sjögren's Disease: Revealing the Connections—a Systematic Review and Meta-Analysis," *Nutrients* 15, no. 3 (January 18, 2023): 497–509, https://doi.org/10.3390/nu15030497.

71. Aduragbemi A. Faniyi et al., "Vitamin D Status and Seroconversion for COVID-19 in UK Healthcare Workers," *The European Respiratory Journal* 2021, no. 57 (December 10, 2020): 2004234, https://doi.org/10.1183/13993003.04234-2020.

72. Christiano Argano et al., "Protective Effect of Vitamin D Supplementation on COVID-19-Related Intensive Care Hospitalization

and Mortality: Definitive Evidence from Meta-Analysis and Trial Sequential Analysis," *Pharmaceuticals* 16, no. 1 (January 16, 2023): 130, https://doi.org/10.3390/ph16010130.

73. The rs ID number (*rs* followed by a number) is the label used in genetic research to identify a specific SNP (single nucleotide polymorphism). SNP indicates that a single nucleotide (adenine, thymine, cytosine, or guanine) in the genome sequence is altered and is present in at least 1 percent of the population.

74. Nicole A. Slater et al., "Genetic Variation in CYP2R1 and GC Genes Associated with Vitamin D Deficiency Status," *Journal of Pharmacy Practice* 30, no. 1 (July 9, 2016): 31, https://doi.org/10.1177/0897190015585876.

Chapter 3

1. John Mellencamp, *Plain Spoken*, recorded September 23, 2014, Republic Records B0021723-02, compact disc.

2. Amanda Petrusich, "John Mellencamp's Mortal Reckoning," *The New Yorker*, January 17, 2022, https://www.newyorker.com/magazine/2022/01/24/john-mellencamps-mortal-reckoning.

3. Lisa J. Pruitt, "Living with Spina Bifida: A Historical Perspective," *Pediatrics* 130, no. 2 (August 1, 2012): 181, https://doi.org/10.1542/peds.2011-2935.

4. "John Mellencamp Meets Doctor Who Saved His Life," CBS Mornings, January 1, 2015, https://www.cbsnews.com/news/john-mellencamp-meets-spina-bifida-doctor-who-saved-his-life/.

5. APNZ, "'Marmageddon' Sends NZ into a Spin," *The New Zealand Herald*, August 15, 2023, https://www.nzherald.co.nz/nz/marmageddon-sends-nz-into-a-spin/DAE6NUTSH2X7AP6TB7VH QYUKWU/.

6. Daphne A. Roe, "Lucy Wills (1888–1964)," *The Journal of Nutrition* 108, no. 9 (September 1, 1978): 1377–83, https://doi.org/10.1093/jn/108.9.1377.

7. H. Bastian, "Lucy Wills (1888–1964): The Life and Research of an Adventurous Independent Woman," *The Journal of the Royal College of Physicians of Edinburgh* 38, no. 1 (April 2008): 90, https://pubmed.ncbi.nlm.nih.gov/19069045/.

8. Lucy Wills, "The Nature of the Hæmopoietic Factor in Marmite," The *Lancet* 221, no. 5729 (June 1, 1933): 1286, https://doi.org/10.1016/s0140-6736(00)85183-1.

9. Sheryl Grant, *Option B: Facing Adversity, Building Resilience, and Finding Joy* (New York: Penguin, 2019).

10. Grant, *Option B*, 17.

11. Chin-Chuan Shih, Yu-Lin Shih, and Jau-Yuan Chen, "The Association between Homocysteine Levels and Cardiovascular Disease Risk among Middle-Aged and Elderly Adults in Taiwan," *BMC Cardiovascular Disorders* 21, no. 1 (April 20, 2021): 191, https://doi.org/10.1186/s12872-021-02000-x.

12. Express News Service, "Nitesh Pandey Heart Attack Death: Why Indian Men in Their 50s Are Most at Risk of Sudden Cardiac Arrest," *The Indian Express*, updated May 25, 2023, https://indianexpress.com/article/health-wellness/nitesh-pandey-death-indian-men-50s-most-at-risk-of-sudden-cardiac-arrest-8627116/.

13. "Report Shows 66% Indians Have Elevated Levels of Homocysteine, Making Them Vulnerable to Heart Diseases; Here's All You Need to Know," *Times of India*, updated April 1, 2023, https://timesofindia.indiatimes.com/life-style/health-fitness/health-news/report-shows-66-indians-have-elevated-levels-of-homocysteine-making-them-vulnerable-to-heart-diseases-heres-all-you-need-to-know/photostory/99165611.cms?from=mdr.

14. Hiroyasu Iso et al., "Serum Total Homocysteine Concentrations and Risk of Stroke and Its Subtypes in Japanese," *Circulation* 109, no. 22 (June 8, 2004): 2766, https://doi.org/10.1161/01.cir.0000131942.77635.2d.

15. Shuai Yuan et al., "Homocysteine, B Vitamins, and Cardiovascular Disease: A Mendelian Randomization Study," *BMC Medicine* 19, no. 1 (April 23, 2021): 97, https://doi.org/10.1186/s12916-021-01977-8.

16. Yanping Li et al., "Folic Acid Supplementation and the Risk of Cardiovascular Diseases: A Meta-Analysis of Randomized Controlled Trials," *Journal of the American Heart Association* 5, no. 8 (August 8, 2016): e003768, https://doi.org/10.1161/jaha.116.003768.

17. Alan D. Kaye et al., "Folic Acid Supplementation in Patients with Elevated Homocysteine Levels," *Advances in Therapy* 37, no. 10 (October 2020): 4159, https://doi.org/10.1007/s12325-020-01474-z.

18. Paul, *The Genetics of Health*, 138.

19. Kaye, "Folic Acid Supplementation in Patients with Elevated Homocysteine Levels."

20. Neetu Tyagi et al., "Mechanisms of Homocysteine-Induced Oxidative Stress," *American Journal of Physiology-Heart and Circulatory Physiology* 289, no. 6 (December 2005): H2649–2656, https://doi.org/10.1152/ajpheart.00548.2005; Byung Jin Kim, Bum Soo Kim, and Jin Ho Kang, "Plasma Homocysteine and Coronary Artery Calcification in Korean Men," *European Journal of Preventive Cardiology* 22, no. 4 (January 30, 2014): 478–85, https://doi.org/10.1177/2047487314522136.

21. Jeong-Min Kim et al., "Relation of Serum Homocysteine Levels to Cerebral Artery Calcification and *Atherosclerosis*," *Atherosclerosis* 254 (November 2016): 200–204, https://doi.org/10.1016/j.atherosclerosis.2016.10.023.

22. Amy B. Karger et al., "Association between Homocysteine and Vascular Calcification Incidence, Prevalence, and Progression in the MESA Cohort," *Journal of the American Heart Association* 9, no. 3 (February 4, 2020): e013934, https://doi .org/10.1161/jaha.119.013934.

23. Susie Jung, Beom-Hee Choi, and Nam-Seok Joo, "Serum Homocysteine and Vascular Calcification: Advances in Mechanisms, Related Diseases, and Nutrition," *Korean Journal of Family Medicine* 43, no. 5 (September 1, 2022): 277–89, https://doi .org/10.4082/kjfm.21.0227.

24. Jacek Baj et al., "Derivatives of Plastics as Potential Carcinogenic Factors: The Current State of Knowledge," *Cancers* 14, no. 19 (2021): 4637, 1–26, https://doi.org/10.3390/cancers14194637.

25. Marte Molenaars et al., "Metabolomics and Lipidomics in Caenorhabditis Elegans Using a Single-Sample Preparation," *Disease Models & Mechanisms* 14, no. 4 (April 1, 2021): 1–12, https://doi.org/10.1242/dmm.047746; Paul, *The Genetics of Health*, 130–131.

26. Andrea Annibal et al., "Regulation of the One Carbon Folate Cycle as a Shared Metabolic Signature of Longevity," *Nature Communications* 12, no. 1 (June 9, 2021):1–14, https://do.orgi /10.1038/s41467-021-23856-9.

27. Annibal et al., "Regulation of the One Carbon Folate Cycle," 4.

28. Filipe Cabreiro et al., "Metformin Retards Aging in C. Elegans by Altering Microbial Folate and Methionine Metabolism," *Cell* 158, no. 1 (March 28, 2013): 228–39, https://doi.org/10.1016 /j.cell.2013.02.035.

29. Chanachai Sae-Lee et al., "Dietary Intervention Modifies DNA Methylation Age Assessed by the Epigenetic Clock," *Molecular Nutrition & Food Research* 62, no. 23 (November 2, 2018): 1800092, https://doi.org/10.1002/mnfr.201800092.

30. Larry A. Tucker, "Serum and Dietary Folate and Vitamin B12 Levels Account for Differences in Cellular Aging: Evidence Based on Telomere Findings in 5581 U.S. Adults," *Oxidative Medicine and Cellular Longevity* 2019 (October 7, 2019): 8, https://doi.org/10.1155/2019/4358717.

31. Tucker, "Serum and Dietary Folate and Vitamin B_{12} Levels Account for Differences in Cellular Aging," 1.

32. Renate M. Winkels et al., "Gender and Body Size Affect the Response of Erythrocyte Folate to Folic Acid Treatment," *The Journal of Nutrition* 138, no. 8 (August 1, 2008): 1456, https://doi.org/10.1093/jn/138.8.1456.

33. Health Canada, "Nutrient Value of Some Common Foods," Government of Canada, 2008, https://www.canada.ca-canada/services/food-nutrition/healthy-eating/en/health/nutrient-data/nutrient-value-some-common-foods-2008.html.

34. Office of Dietary Supplements, "Choline: Fact Sheet for Health Professionals," National Institutes of Health, accessed December 20, 2023, https://ods.od.nih.gov/factsheets/Choline-HealthProfessional/#h3.

Chapter 4

1. Gary Beauchamp, "The Flavor of Serendipity," *American Scientist* 107, no. 3 (May–June 2019): 170, https://doi.org/10.1511/2019.107.3.170.

2. Beauchamp, "The Flavor of Serendipity."

3. F. Gutierrez-Rosales, José Julián Ríos, and Ma L Gomez-Rey, "Main Polyphenols in the Bitter Taste of Virgin Olive Oil. Structural Confirmation by On-Line High-Performance Liquid Chromatography Electrospray Ionization Mass Spectrometry,"

Journal of Agricultural and Food Chemistry 51, no. 20 (August 29, 2003): 6024, https://doi.org/10.1021/jf021199x.

4. Gary K. Beauchamp et al.,"Ibuprofen-Like Activity in Extra-Virgin Olive Oil," *Nature* 437, no. 7055 (August 31, 2005): 45, https://doi.org/10.1038/437045a.

5. Lorenzo Flori et al., "The Nutraceutical Value of Olive Oil and Its Bioactive Constituents on the Cardiovascular System. Focusing on Main Strategies to Slow Down Its Quality Decay during Production and Storage," *Nutrients* 11, no. 9 (September 2019): 1962, https://doi.org/10.3390/nu11091962.

6. Flori, "The Nutraceutical Value of Olive Oil and Its Bioactive Constituents on the Cardiovascular System," 1962.

7. Antonio Segura-Carretero and Jose Antonio Curiel, "Current Disease-Targets for Oleocanthal as Promising Natural Therapeutic Agent," *International Journal of Molecular Sciences* 19, no. 10 (October 2018): 2899, 3, https://doi.org/10.3390/ijms19102899.

8. Beatrice Polini et al.,"Oleocanthal and Oleacein Contribute to the in Vitro Therapeutic Potential of Extra Virgin Oil-Derived Extracts in Non-Melanoma Skin Cancer," *Toxicology in Vitro: An International Journal Published in Association with BIBRA* 52 (October 1, 2018): 243, https://doi.org/10.1016/j.tiv.2018.06.021.

9. Nehad M. Ayoub et al., "The Olive Oil Phenolic (-)-Oleocanthal Modulates Estrogen Receptor Expression in Luminal Breast Cancer in Vitro and in Vivo and Synergizes with Tamoxifen Treatment," *European Journal of Pharmacology* 810 (September 5, 2017): 100, https://doi.org/10.1016/j.ejphar.2017.06.019.

10. Yazan S. Batarseh and Amal Kaddoumi, "Oleocanthal-Rich Extra-Virgin Olive Oil Enhances Donepezil Effect by Reducing Amyloid-β Load and Related Toxicity in a Mouse Model of

Alzheimer's Disease," *The Journal of Nutritional Biochemistry* 55 (May 2018): 113, https://doi.org/10.1016/j.jnutbio.2017.12.006.

11. R. W. Owen et al., "Phenolic Compounds and Squalene in Olive Oils: The Concentration and Antioxidant Potential of Total Phenols, Simple Phenols, Secoiridoids, Lignansand Squalene," *Food and Chemical Toxicology* 38, no. 8 (August 2000): 647, https://doi.org/10.1016/s0278-6915(00)00061-2.

12. Antonio Segura-Carretero and Jose Antonio Curiel, "Current Disease-Targets for Oleocanthal as Promising Natural Therapeutic Agent," *International Journal of Molecular Sciences* 19, no. 10 (October 1, 2018): 2899, https://doi.org/10.3390/ijms19102899.

13. Josiemer Mattei et al., "TCF7L2 Genetic Variants Modulate the Effect of Dietary Fat Intake on Changes in Body Composition during a Weight-Loss Intervention," *The American Journal of Clinical Nutrition* 96, no. 5 (November 1, 2012): 1129, https://doi.org/10.3945/ajcn.112.038125.

14. Nithya Neelakantan, Jowy Yi Hoong Seah, and Rob M. van Dam, "The Effect of Coconut Oil Consumption on Cardiovascular Risk Factors: A Systematic Review and Meta-Analysis of Clinical Trials," *Circulation* 141, no. 10 (January 13, 2020): 804, https://doi.org/10.1161/circulationaha.119.043052.

15. Neelakantan, Seah, and van Dam, "The Effect of Coconut Oil Consumption on Cardiovascular Risk Factors," 812.

16. Health Canada, "Nutrient Value of Some Common Foods."

17. Ronald P. Mensink et al., "Effects of Dietary Fatty Acids and Carbohydrates on the Ratio of Serum Total to HDL Cholesterol and on Serum Lipids and Apolipoproteins: A Meta-Analysis of 60 Controlled Trials," *The American Journal of Clinical Nutrition* 77, no. 5 (May 2003): 1146–55, https://doi.org/10.1093/ajcn/77.5.1146.

18. Dolores Corella, "APOA2, Dietary Fat, and Body Mass Index," *Archives of Internal Medicine* 169, no. 20 (November 9, 2009): 1897, https://doi.org/10.1001/archinternmed.2009.343.

19. Gisele K. Rodrigues et al., "A Single FTO Gene Variant Rs9939609 Is Associated with Body Weight Evolution in a Multiethnic Extremely Obese Population That Underwent Bariatric Surgery," *Nutrition* 31, no. 11–12 (November 2015): 1344–50, https://doi .org/10.1016/j.nut.2015.05.020.

20. Health Canada, "Nutrient Value of Some Common Foods."

21. Jeremy D. Furtado et al., "Pharmacological Inhibition of CETP (Cholesteryl Ester Transfer Protein) Increases HDL (High-Density Lipoprotein) That Contains ApoC3 and Other HDL Subspecies Associated with Higher Risk of Coronary Heart Disease," *Arteriosclerosis, Thrombosis, and Vascular Biology* 42, no. 2 (December 23, 2022): 227, https://doi.org/10.1161/atvbaha.121.317181.

22. Philip J. Barter et al., "Effects of Torcetrapib in Patients at High Risk for Coronary Events," *New England Journal of Medicine* 357, no. 21 (November 22, 2007): 2109, https://doi.org/10.1056/nejmoa0706628.

23. Chang Liu et al., "Association between High-Density Lipoprotein Cholesterol Levels and Adverse Cardiovascular Outcomes in High-Risk Populations," *JAMA Cardiology* 7, no. 7 (May 18, 2022): 672, https://doi.org/10.1001/jamacardio.2022.0912.

24. Dennis T. Ko et al., "High-Density Lipoprotein Cholesterol and Cause-Specific Mortality in Individuals without Previous Cardiovascular Conditions: The CANHEART Study," *Journal of the American College of Cardiology* 68, no. 19 (November 8, 2016): 2073, https://doi.org/10.1016/j.jacc.2016.08.038.

25. Min-Gyu Yoo et al., "The Effect of the Association between CETP Variant Type and Alcohol Consumption on Cholesterol Level Differs according to the ALDH2 Variant Type,"

Scientific Reports 12, no. 1 (September 6, 2022): 15129, https://doi .org/10.1038/s41598-022-19171-y.

26. Fabrizia Bonacina et al., 2021. "HDL in Immune-Inflammatory Responses: Implications Beyond Cardiovascular Diseases," *Cells* 10, no. 5 (April 29, 2021): 1061, https://doi.org/10.3390 /cells10051061.

27. Harrison Wein, "When HDL Cholesterol Doesn't Protect against Heart Disease," National Institutes of Health (NIH), March 21, 2016, https:// www.nih.gov/news-events/nih-research-matters /when-hdl-cholesterol-doesnt-protect-against-heart-disease.

28. Yasser Nassef et al., "Association between Aerobic Exercise and High-Density Lipoprotein Cholesterol Levels across Various Ranges of Body Mass Index and Waist-Hip Ratio and the Modulating Role of the Hepatic Lipase Rs1800588 Variant," *Genes* 10, no. 6 (June 10, 2019): 440, https://doi.org/10.3390 /genes10060440.

29. Gordon S. Huggins et al., "Do Genetic Modifiers of High-Density Lipoprotein Cholesterol and Triglyceride Levels Also Modify Their Response to a Lifestyle Intervention in the Setting of Obesity and Type-2 Diabetes Mellitus?" *Circulation: Cardiovascular Genetics* 6, no. 4 (August 2013): 391, https://doi.org/10.1161 /circgenetics.113.000042.

30. Huggins, "Do Genetic Modifiers of High-Density Lipoprotein Cholesterol and Triglyceride Levels Also Modify Their Response to a Lifestyle Intervention in the Setting of Obesity and Type-2 Diabetes Mellitus?" 396.

31. Yingchang Lu et al.,"Dietary N–3 and N–6 Polyunsaturated Fatty Acid Intake Interacts with FADS1 Genetic Variation to Affect Total and HDL-Cholesterol Concentrations in the Doetinchem Cohort Study," *The American Journal of Clinical Nutrition* 92, no. 1 (May 19, 2010): 258, https://doi .org/10.3945/ajcn.2009.29130.

32. Health Canada, "Canadian Nutrient File (CNF)—Search by Food," Government of Canada, accessed July 21, 2024, https://food-nutrition.canada.ca/cnf-fce.

33. Zhen He et al., "FADS1-FADS2 Genetic Polymorphisms Are Associated with Fatty Acid Metabolism through Changes in DNA Methylation and Gene Expression," *Clinical Epigenetics* 10, no. 1, (August 29, 2018): 1, https://doi.org/10.1186/s13148-018-0545-5.

34. Yingchang Lu et al., "Dietary N–3 and N–6 Polyunsaturated Fatty Acid Intake Interacts with FADS1 Genetic Variation to Affect Total and HDL-Cholesterol Concentrations in the Doetinchem Cohort Study," *The American Journal of Clinical Nutrition* 92, no. 1 (July 2010): 258–65, https://doi.org/10.3945/ajcn.2009.29130.

35. The word *elaidic* has origins in the French name for it, *acide élaidique* ("acid similar to olive oil"), which is what Boudet called it when he isolated this eighteen-carbon fatty acid in the lab: "Elaidic Acid: Structure, Properties, and Food Sources," Tuscany Diet, accessed February 10, 2024, https://www.tuscany-diet.net/lipids/fatty-acids/elaidic-acid.

36. A. Aro, "Fatty Acids | Trans-fatty Acids: Health Effects," *Encyclopedia of Food Sciences and Nutrition (Second Edition)*, ed. Benjamin Caballero (Cambridge, MA: Academic Press, 2003): 2324–30, https://doi.org/10.1016/B0-12-227055-X/01365-1.

37. Kalyana Sundram, "Trans (Elaidic) Fatty Acids Adversely Affect the Lipoprotein Profile Relative to Specific Saturated Fatty Acids in Humans," *The Journal of Nutrition* 127, no. 3 (March 1, 1997): 514S520S, https://doi.org/10.1093/jn/127.3.514s.

38. Robert A. Norman and Sharad P. Paul, *The Last Natural Man* (New York: Springer International Publishing, 2017).

39. Adiv A. Johnson et al., "The Role of DNA Methylation in Aging, Rejuvenation, and Age-Related Disease," *Rejuvenation*

Research 15, no. 5 (October 2012): 483, https://doi.org/10.1089/rej.2012.1324.

40. Giovanni Fiorito et al., "DNA Methylation-Based Biomarkers of Aging Were Slowed down in a Two-Year Diet and Physical Activity Intervention Trial: The DAMA Study," *Aging Cell* 20, no. 10 (October 1, 2021): e13439, https://doi.org/10.1111/acel.13439.

41. José Flores-Sierra et al., "The Trans Fatty Acid Elaidate Affects the Global DNA Methylation Profile of Cultured Cells and in Vivo," *Lipids in Health and Disease* 15 (April 12, 2016): 75, https://doi.org/10.1186/s12944-016-0243-2.

42. Véronique Chajès et al., "Plasma Elaidic Acid Level as Biomarker of Industrial Trans Fatty Acids and Risk of Weight Change: Report from the EPIC Study," *PLOS ONE* 10, no. 2 (February 12, 2015): e0118206, https://doi.org/10.1371/journal.pone.0118206.

43. Nathalie Michels et al., "Dietary Trans-Fatty Acid Intake in Relation to Cancer Risk: A Systematic Review and Meta-Analysis," *Nutrition Reviews* 79, no. 7 (November 3, 2020): 758, https://doi.org/10.1093/nutrit/nuaa061.

44. "Trans-Fatty Acids," Pan American Health Organization, World Health Organization, accessed February 11, 2024, https://www.paho.org/en/topics/trans-fatty-acids.

45. Vandana Dhaka et al., "Trans Fats—Sources, Health Risks and Alternative Approach—A Review," *Journal of Food Science and Technology* 48, no. 5 (January 28, 2011): 534, https://doi.org/10.1007/s13197-010-0225-8.

46. Jorge Salmerón et al., "Dietary Fat Intake and Risk of Type 2 Diabetes in Women," *The American Journal of Clinical Nutrition* 73, no. 6 (June 1, 2001): 1023, https://doi.org/10.1093/ajcn/73.6.1019.

47. Takanori Honda et al., "Serum Elaidic Acid Concentration and Risk of Dementia," *Neurology* (October 2019): e2053–64, https://doi.org/10.1212/wnl.0000000000008464.

48. Malathy Sriram, "The Dalda Story," *BusinessLine on Campus*, April 16, 2016, https://bloncampus.thehindubusinessline.com /columns/brand-basics/the-dalda-story/article8462248.ece.

49. Outlook Web Desk, "It's Time to Bid Goodbye to Vanaspati," Outlook Publishing India Pvt Ltd, December 2, 2022, https:// planet.outlookindia.com/opinions/it-s-time-to-bid-goodbye-to -vanaspati-news-413586.

50. Nutrition and Food Safety, "Replace Trans Fat: AN Action Package to Eliminate Industrially Produced Trans-Fatty Acids," World Health Organization, May 2021, https://www .who.int/publications/i/item/9789240021105.

51. Parmita Uniyal, "Killer Trans Fats: How Samosa and French Fries are Damaging Your Heart; List of Foods With Trans Fats You Should Skip," *Hindustan Times*, August 16, 2023, https:// www.hindustantimes.com/lifestyle/health/killer-trans-fats-how -samosa-and-french-fries-are-damaging-your-heart-list-of -foods-with-trans-fats-you-should-skip-101692166441175.html.

52. Marta Garaulet et al., "PPARγ Pro12Ala Interacts with Fat Intake for Obesity and Weight Loss in a Behavioural Treatment Based on the Mediterranean Diet," *Molecular Nutrition & Food Research* 55, no. 12 (November 21, 2011): 1771, https://doi.org/10.1002 /mnfr.201100437.

53. N. Shaat et al., "A Variant in the Transcription Factor 7-like 2 (TCF7L2) Gene Is Associated with an Increased Risk of Gestational Diabetes Mellitus," *Diabetologia* 50, no. 5 (March 7, 2007): 972–79, https://doi.org/10.1007/s00125-007-0623-2.

54. Katrine Grau et al., "TCF7L2 Rs7903146–Macronutrient Interaction in Obese Individuals' Responses to a 10-Wk Randomized Hypoenergetic Diet," *The American Journal of Clinical Nutrition* 91, no. 2 (February 1, 2010): 475, https://doi.org/10.3945/ajcn .2009.27947.

55. Health Canada, "Nutrient Value of Some Common Foods."

Chapter 5

1. John Yudkin, *Pure, White, and Deadly* (London: Davis-Poynter, 1972).

2. John Yudkin, "Patterns and Trends in Carbohydrate Consumption and Their Relation to Disease," *Proceedings of the Nutrition Society* 23, no. 2 (September 1964): 149, https://doi.org/10.1079/pns19640028.

3. Yudkin, "Patterns and Trends in Carbohydrate Consumption and Their Relation to Disease," 160.

4. Yudkin, "Patterns and Trends in Carbohydrate Consumption and Their Relation to Disease," 160.

5. Ancel Keys, "Sucrose in the Diet and Coronary Heart Disease," *Atherosclerosis* 14, no. 2 (September 1971): 193, https://doi.org/10.1016/0021-9150(71)90049-9.

6. Robert H. Lustig, "Sugar: The Bitter Truth," interview by University of California Television, July 30, 2009, video, 1:29:36, July 30, 2009, https://www.youtube.com/watch?v=dBnniua6-oM.

7. Lustig, "Sugar: The Bitter Truth," 0:18.40–0:18.43.

8. Lustig, "Sugar: The Bitter Truth," 0:18.51–20.00.

9. Tom Sasse and Sophie Metcalfe, "Sugar Tax," *Institute for Government*, November 14, 2022, https://www.instituteforgovernment.org.uk/article/explainer/sugar-tax.

10. Sharad Paul, "Genes, Germs and Geography: The Future of Medicine" (lecture, Chatham House, London, April 24, 2018), accessed October 2022, https://www.chathamhouse.org/archive/genes-germs-and-geography-future-medicine.

11. Rebecca K. Kelly et al., "Associations between Types and Sources of Dietary Carbohydrates and Cardiovascular Disease Risk: A Prospective Cohort Study of UK Biobank Participants," *BMC*

Medicine 21, no. 1 (February 14, 2023): 1, https://doi.org/10.1186/s12916-022-02712-7.

12. Kelly et al., "Associations between Types and Sources of Dietary Carbohydrates and Cardiovascular Disease Risk," 3.

13. "Get the Facts: Added Sugars," Nutrition, US Centers for Disease Control and Prevention, January 5, 2024, https://www.cdc.gov/nutrition/php/data-research/added-sugars.html?CDC_AAref_Val=https://www.cdc.gov/nutrition/data-statistics/added-sugars.html.

14. James M. Rippe and Theodore J. Angelopoulos, "Sucrose, High-Fructose Corn Syrup, and Fructose, Their Metabolism and Potential Health Effects: What Do We Really Know?" *Advances in Nutrition* 4, no. 2 (March 2013): 238, https://doi.org/10.3945/an.112.002824.

15. Marsha M. Wheeler and Gene E. Robinson, "Diet-Dependent Gene Expression in Honey Bees: Honey Vs. Sucrose or High Fructose Corn Syrup," *Scientific Reports* 4, 5726 (July 17, 2014), https://doi.org/10.1038/srep05726.

16. S. Boyd Eaton, "The Ancestral Human Diet: What Was It and Should It Be a Paradigm for Contemporary Nutrition?" *Proceedings of the Nutrition Society* 65, no. 1 (February 2006): 1, https://doi.org/10.1079/pns2005471.

17. Kushagra Mathur et al., "Effect of Artificial Sweeteners on Insulin Resistance Among Type-2 Diabetes Mellitus Patients," *Journal of Family Medicine and Primary Care* 9, no. 1 (January 28, 2020): 69, https://doi.org/10.4103/jfmpc.jfmpc_329_19.

18. Charlotte Debras et al., "Artificial Sweeteners and Risk of Cardiovascular Diseases: Results from the Prospective NutriNet-Santé Cohort," *BMJ* 378, no. 8351 (September 7, 2022): e071204, https://doi.org/10.1136/bmj-2022-071204.

19. Miryam Naddaf, "Aspartame Is a Possible Carcinogen: The Science behind the Decision," *Nature*, July 14, 2023, https://doi.org/10.1038/d41586-023-02306-0.

20. Sandeep Singh et al., "The Contentious Relationship between Artificial Sweeteners and Cardiovascular Health," *The Egyptian Journal of Internal Medicine* 35, no. 1 (June 20, 2023): 1–6, https://doi.org/10.1186/s43162-023-00232-1.

21. Yantong Meng et al., "Sugar- and Artificially Sweetened Beverages Consumption Linked to Type 2 Diabetes, Cardiovascular Diseases, and All-Cause Mortality: A Systematic Review and Dose-Response Meta-Analysis of Prospective Cohort Studies," *Nutrients* 13, no. 8 (July 30, 2021): 2636, https://doi.org/10.3390/nu13082636.

22. Marco Witkowski et al., "The Artificial Sweetener Erythritol and Cardiovascular Event Risk," *Nature Medicine* 29 (February 27, 2023): 710, https://doi.org/10.1038/s41591-023-02223-9.

23. Jotham Suez et al., "Personalized Microbiome-Driven Effects of Non-Nutritive Sweeteners on Human Glucose Tolerance," *Cell* 185, no. 18 (August 17, 2022): 3307, https://doi.org/10.1016/j.cell.2022.07.016.

24. Zoe Diana Draelos, "Aging Skin: The Role of Diet: Facts and Controversies," *Clinics in Dermatology* 31, no. 6 (November 2013): 703, https://doi.org/10.1016/j.clindermatol.2013.05.005.

25. Raitis Pečulis et al., "Identification of Glyoxalase 1 Polymorphisms Associated with Enzyme Activity," *Gene* 515, no. 1 (February 1, 2013): 140, https://doi.org/10.1016/j.gene.2012.11.009.

26. Gemma Aragonès et al., "The Glyoxalase System in Age-Related Diseases: Nutritional Intervention as Anti-Ageing Strategy," *Cells* 10, no. 8 (July 2021): 1852, https://doi.or/10.3390/cells10081852.

27. Peter Schuck, "Glycated Hemoglobin as a Physiological Measure of Stress and Its Relations to Some Psychological Stress Indica-

tors," *Behavioral Medicine* 24, no. 2 (January 1998): 93, https://doi.org/10. 1080/08964289809596386.

28. Karla E. Merz and Debbie C. Thurmond, "Role of Skeletal Muscle in Insulin Resistance and Glucose Uptake," *Comprehensive Physiology* 10 no. 3 (July 2020): 785, https://doi.org/10.1002/cphy.c190029.

29. Bianca M. J. Martens et al., "Amylopectin Structure and Crystallinity Explains Variation in Digestion Kinetics of Starches across Botanic Sources in an in Vitro Pig Model," *Journal of Animal Science and Biotechnology* 9, no. 1 (December 29, 2018): 2, https://doi.org/10.1186/s40104-018-0303-8.

30. Marilyn C. Cornelis et al., "TCF7L2, Dietary Carbohydrate, and Risk of Type 2 Diabetes in US Women," *The American Journal of Clinical Nutrition* 89, no. 4 (February 11, 2009): 1256, https://doi.org/10.3945/ajcn.2008.27058.

31. Y.-J. Choi et al., "Association between Salivary Amylase (AMY1) Gene Copy Numbers and Insulin Resistance in Asymptomatic Korean Men," *Diabetic Medicine* 32, no. 12 (May 20, 2015): 1588, https://doi.org/10.1111/dme.12808; Paul, *The Genetics of Health*, 195.

32. Karen M. Eny et al.,"Genetic Variant in the Glucose Transporter Type 2 Is Associated with Higher Intakes of Sugars in Two Distinct Populations," *Physiological Genomics* 33, no. 3 (May 1, 2008): 355, https://doi.org/10.1152/physiolgenomics.00148.2007.

33. Linda Eriksson et al., "Allelic Variation in Taste Genes Is Associated with Taste and Diet Preferences and Dental Caries," *Nutrients* 11, no. 7 (June 29, 2019): 1491, https://doi.org/10.3390/nu11071491.

34. G. V. Kulkarni et al., "Association of GLUT2 and TAS1R2 Genotypes with Risk for Dental Caries," *Caries Research* 47, no. 3 (April 2013): 219, https://doi.org/10.1159/000345652.

35. Health Canada, "Nutrient Value of Some Common Foods."

36. "WHO Calls on Countries to Reduce Sugars Intake Among Adults and Children," *World Health Organization* (March 4, 2015): https://www.who.int/news/item/04-03-2015-who-calls-on-countries-to-reduce-sugars-intake-among-adults-and-children.

37. Health Canada, "Nutrient Value of Some Common Foods."

38. Courtney Nguyen, "Andy Roddick Nearly Came to Blows with Novak Djokovic after '08 U.S. Open Loss," *Sports Illustrated*, October 3, 2013, https://www.si.com/tennis/2013/10/03/andy-roddick-novak-djokovic-fighting-2008-us-open.

39. Chris Oddo, "By the Numbers: Djokovic's four US Open & 24 Grand Slam Titles," Us Open, September 10, 2023, https://www.usopen.org/en_US/news/articles/2023-09-10/by_the_numbers_djokovics_four_us_open_24_grand_slam_titles.html.

40. Jordan Sanford, "Eat to Win: Novak Djokovic Reveals More about His Gluten-Free Diet," *Tennis*, February 18, 2022, https://www.tennis.com/baseline/articles/eat-to-win-novak-djokovic-reveals-more-about-gluten-free-diet-bbc-interview.

41. Paul, *The Genetics of Health*, 197.

42. Hugh J. Freeman, "Celiac Disease Assocaited with Primary Biliary Cirrhosis in a Coast Salish Native," *Canadian Journal of Gastroenterology* 8, no. 2 (1994): 105, https://doi.org/10.1155/1994/150426.

43. E. J. Hall and R. M. Batt, "Dietary Modulation of Gluten Sensitivity in a Naturally Occurring Enteropathy of Irish Setter Dogs," *Gut* 33, no. 2 (February 1992): 198, https://doi.org/10.1136/gut.33.2.198.

44. Gursimran Singh Kochhar et al., "Celiac Disease: Managing a Multisystem Disorder," *Cleveland Clinic Journal of Medicine* 83, no. 3 (March 1, 2016): 217, https://doi.org/10.3949/ccjm.83a.14158.

45. Benjamin Lebwohl, Jonas F Ludvigsson, and Peter H. R. Green, "Celiac Disease and Non-Celiac Gluten Sensitivity," *British Medi-*

cal Journal 351 (October 5, 2015): h4347, https://doi.org/10.1136/bmj.h4347.

46. The Lancet Gastroenterology & Hepatology, "Gluten: Going against the Grain?" *The Lancet Gastroenterology & Hepatology* 1, no. 2 (October 2016): 85, https://doi.org/10.1016/s2468-1253(16)30087-5.

47. Novak Djokovic, *Serve to Win* (New York: Zinc Ink, 2013).

48. Louis A. Duhring, "Dermatitis Herpetiformis," *JAMA* III, no. 9 (August 30, 1884): 225, https://doi.org/10.1001/jama.1884.02390580001001.

49. Kelly Servick, "What's Really behind 'Gluten Sensitivity'?" *Science*, May 23, 2018, https://www.science.org/content/article/what-s-really-behind -gluten-sensitivity.

50. Jacqueline S. Barrett, "How to Institute the Low-FODMAP Diet," *Journal of Gastroenterology and Hepatology* 32, no. S1 (February 28, 2017): 8–10, https://doi.org/10.1111/jgh.13686.

51. Victorien M. Wolters and Cisca Wijmenga, "Genetic Background of Celiac Disease and Its Clinical Implications," *The American Journal of Gastroenterology* 103, no. 1 (January 1, 2008): 190, https://doi.org/10.1111/j.1572-0241.2007.01471.x.

52. Michele Sallese et al., "Beyond the HLA Genes in Gluten-Related Disorders," *Frontiers in Nutrition* 7 (November 12, 2020): 2, https://doi.org/10.3389/fnut.2020.575844.

53. Veronica Bonciolini et al., "Cutaneous Manifestations of Non-Celiac Gluten Sensitivity: Clinical Histological and Immunopathological Features," *Nutrients* 7, no. 9 (September 15, 2015): 7798, https://doi.org/10.3390/nu7095368.

54. Christian Juhl et al., "Dairy Intake and Acne Vulgaris: A Systematic Review and Meta-Analysis of 78,529 Children, Adolescents, and Young Adults," *Nutrients* 10, no. 8 (August 9, 2018): 1049, https://doi.org/10.3390/nu10081049.

55. Clement A. Adebamowo et al., "High School Dietary Dairy Intake and Teenage Acne," *Journal of the American Academy of Dermatology* 52, no. 2 (February 2005): 207–14, https://doi .org/10.1016/j.jaad.2004.08.007.

56. Liliane Laure Toukam et al., "In Vivo Antimalarial Activity of a Probiotic bacterium Lactobacillus sakei Isolated from Traditionally Fermented Milk in BALB/c Mice Infected with Plasmodium berghei ANKA," *Journal of Ethnopharmacology* 280 (November 15, 2021): 114448, https://doi.org/10.1016/j.jep.2021.114448.

57. Cecilie Siggaard Jørgensen et al., "Milk Products in the Treatment of Hypophosphatemic Rickets: A Pilot Study," *International Journal of Endocrinology and Metabolism* 17, no. 4 (October 6, 2019): 1, https://doi.org/10.5812/ijem.91454.

58. T. Sahi, "Genetics and Epidemiology of Adult-Type Hypolactasia," *Scandinavian Journal of Gastroenterology* 29, no. sup202 (1994): 7, https://doi.org/10.3109/00365529409091740.

59. P. Gerbault et al., "Evolution of Lactase Persistence: An Example of Human Niche Construction," *Philosophical Transactions of the Royal Society B: Biological Sciences* 366, no. 1566 (March 27, 2011): 863, https://doi.org/10.1098/rstb.2010.0268.

60. J. Ji, J. Sundquist, and K. Sundquist, "Lactose Intolerance and Risk of Lung, Breast and Ovarian Cancers: Aetiological Clues from a Population-Based Study in Sweden," *British Journal of Cancer* 112, no. 1 (October 14, 2014): 149, https://doi.org/10.1038 /bjc.2014.544.

61. Ethel-Michele de Villiers and Harald zur Hausen, "Bovine Meat and Milk Factors (BMMFs): Their Proposed Role in Common Human Cancers and Type 2 Diabetes Mellitus," *Cancers* 13, no. 21 (October 28, 2021): 5407; 1, https://doi.org/10.3390 /cancers13215407.

62. "Harald zur Hausen," The Nobel Prize, accessed February 23, 2024, https://www.nobelprize.org/prizes/medicine/2008/hausen/facts/.

63. de Villiers and zur Hausen, "Bovine Meat and Milk Factors," 1.

64. "Breast Cancer in New Zealand," Breast Cancer Foundation NZ, accessed May 21, 2024, https://www.breastcancerfoundation.org.nz/breast-awareness/breast-cancer-facts/breast-cancer-in-nz.

65. Sridhar Alla and Deborah F. Mason, "Multiple Sclerosis in New Zealand," *Journal of Clinical Neuroscience* 21, no. 8 (2014): 1288, https://doi.org/10.1016/j.jocn.2013.09.009.

66. Brett J. Wade, "Spatial Analysis of Global Prevalence of Multiple Sclerosis Suggests Need for an Updated Prevalence Scale," *Multiple Sclerosis International* 2014, no. 1 (January 2014): 2, https://doi.org/10.1155/2014/124578.

67. "In 2015, Every Israeli Consumed an Average of 1 Liter of Milk per Week," Ministry of Agriculture and Food Security, Government of Israel, September 6, 2016, https://www.gov.il/en/pages/2015milk.

68. Zbigniew Dzialanski et al., "Lactase Persistence versus Lactose Intolerance: Is There an Intermediate Phenotype?" *Clinical Biochemistry* 49, no. 3 (February 2016): 248–52, https://doi.org/10.1016/j.clinbiochem.2015.11.001.

69. W. Nadia H. Koek et al., "The T-13910C Polymorphism in the Lactase Phlorizin Hydrolase Gene Is Associated with Differences in Serum Calcium Levels and Calcium Intake," *Journal of Bone and Mineral Research* 25, no. 9 (September 1, 2010): 1980, https://doi.org/10.1002/jbmr.83.

70. Adebamowo et al., "High School Dietary Dairy Intake and Teenage Acne," 207–14.

71. Joseph Francis De Luca et al., "Goat Milk Skin Products May Cause the Development of Goat Milk Allergy," *Clinical &*

Experimental Allergy 52, no. 5 (April 6, 2022): 706, https://doi.org/10.1111/cea.14133.

72. "What Is the Lactose Content of Different Dairy Products?" Dairy Australia, updated July 3, 2024, https://www.dairy.com.au/dairy-matters/you-ask-we-answer/what-is-the-lactose-content-of-different-dairy-products.

73. "Surviving in Salt Water," American Museum of Natural History, accessed May 20, 2024, https://www.amnh.org/exhibitions/water-h2o--life/life-in-water/surviving-in-salt-water.

74. "Facts and Ideas from Anywhere," *Baylor University Medical Center Proceedings* 14, no. 3 (July 2001): 314, https://www.ncbi.nlm.nih.gov/pm/articles/PMC1305840/.

75. L. Tobian, "Salt and Hypertension. Lessons from Animal Models That Relate to Human Hypertension," *Hypertension* 17, no. 1 (January 1, 1991): I52, https://doi.org/10.1161/01.hyp.17.1_suppl.i52.

76. Feng J. He, Sonia Pombo-Rodrigues, and Graham A. MacGregor, "Salt Reduction in England from 2003 to 2011: Its Relationship to Blood Pressure, Stroke and Ischaemic Heart Disease Mortality," *BMJ Open* 4, no. 4 (April 2014): e004549, https://doi.org/10.1136/bmjopen-2013-004549.

77. Kirsten Bibbins-Domingo et al., "Projected Effect of Dietary Salt Reductions on Future Cardiovascular Disease," *New England Journal of Medicine* 362, no. 7 (February 18, 2010): 590–99, https://doi.org/10.1056/nejmoa0907355.

78. Bibbins-Domingo, "Projected Effect of Dietary Salt Reductions on Future Cardiovascular Disease," 590.

79. Graham H. MacGregor, H E de Wardener, "Commentary: Salt, Blood Pressure and Health," *International Journal of Epidemiology* 31, no. 2, (April 2002): 322, https://doi.org/10.1093/ije/31.2.320.

80. MacGregor and de Wardener, "Commentary: Salt, Blood Pressure and Health," 325.

81. Djin Liem, "Infants' and Children's Salt Taste Perception and Liking: A Review," *Nutrients* 9, no. 9 (September 13, 2017): 1011, https://doi.org/10.3390/nu9091011.

82. Better Health Channel, "Salt," Department of Health, State Government of Victoria, Australia, reviewed June 23, 2022, https://www.betterhealth.vic.gov.au/health/healthyliving/salt#.

83. "Where's the Salt?" *Harvard Public Health Magazine*, July 28, 2016, https://www.hsph.harvard.edu/magazine/magazine_article/wheres-the-salt/.

84. "Taste and Flavor Roles of Sodium in Foods: A Unique Challenge to Reducing Sodium Intake," in *Institute of Medicine (US) Committee on Strategies to Reduce Sodium Intake*, Jane E. Henney, Christine L. Taylor, and Caitlin S. Boon, eds. (Washington, DC: National Academies Press, 2010), https://www.ncbi.nlm.nih.gov/books/NBK50958/.

85. Esteban Poch et al., "Molecular Basis of Salt Sensitivity in Human Hypertension," *Hypertension* 38, no. 5 (November 2001): 1204, https://doi.org/10.1161/hy1101.099479.

86. Tuba Gunel et al., "Comparison of Elite Athletes and Essential Hypertension Patients for *Angiotensin-Converting Enzyme (ACE)* I/D and ACE G2350A Gene Polymorphisms," *Biomedical Journal of Scientific & Technical Research* 31, no. 1 (October 2020): 23829, https://doi.org/10.26717/bjstr.2020.31.005032.

87. Office of Disease Prevention and Health Promotion, "Eat Less Sodium: Quick Tips," US Department of Health and Human Services, updated August 22, 2023, https://health.gov/myhealthfinder/health-conditions/heart-health/eat-less-sodium-quick-tips.

88. Health Canada, "Nutrient Value of Some Common Foods."

Chapter 6

1. *The Sound of Music*, directed by Robert Wise, starring Julie Andrews (1965; Los Angeles, CA: 20th Century Fox, 2015), DVD.

2. "The Don't Worry Movement.; Its Father, Theodore Frelinghuysen Seward, Speaks of Its Principles," *New York Times*, February 27, 1898, https://www.nytimes.com/1898/02/27/archives/the-dont-worry-movement-its-father-theodore-frelinghuysen-seward.html.

3. Kelly McGonigal, *The Upside of Stress: Why Stress Is Good for You, and How to Get Good at It* (New York: Avery Publishing, 2015).

4. Abiola Keller et al., "Does the Perception That Stress Affects Health Matter? The Association with Health and Mortality," *Health Psychology* 31, no. 5 (2012): 677, https://doi.org/10.1037/a0026743.

5. Keller et al., "Does the Perception That Stress Affects Health Matter?" 677.

6. Timothy J. Schoenfeld and Elizabeth Gould, "Stress, Stress Hormones, and Adult Neurogenesis," *Experimental Neurology* 233, no. 1 (January 2012): 12, https://doi.org/10.1016/j.expneurol.2011.01.008.

7. Firdaus S. Dhabhar, "The Short-Term Stress Response—Mother Nature's Mechanism for Enhancing Protection and Performance under Conditions of Threat, Challenge, and Opportunity," *Frontiers in Neuroendocrinology* 49 (April 2018): 175, https://doi.org/10.1016/j.yfrne.2018.03.004.

8. Janet A. DiPietro et al., "Maternal Psychological Distress during Pregnancy in Relation to Child Development at Age Two," *Child Development* 77, no. 3 (May 2006): 573, https://doi.org/10.1111/j.1467-8624.2006.00891.x.

9. Margaret Johnstone and Ainsley Johnstone, *Living with a Black Dog* (London: Robinson, 2008).

10. Marcel Ebrecht et al., "Perceived Stress and Cortisol Levels Predict Speed of Wound Healing in Healthy Male Adults," *Psycho neuroendocrinology* 29, no. 6 (July 2004): 798, https://doi.org/10.1016/s0306-4530(03)00144-6.

11. Hilary A. Tindle et al., "Optimism, Cynical Hostility, and Incident Coronary Heart Disease and Mortality in the Women's Health Initiative," *Circulation* 120, no. 8 (August 25, 2009): 660, https://doi.org/10.1161/circulationaha.108.827642.

12. Erik J. Giltay et al., "Dispositional Optimism and All-Cause and Cardiovascular Mortality Ina Prospective Cohort of Elderly Dutch Men and Women," *Archives of General Psychiatry* 61, no. 11 (November 1, 2004): 1126, https://doi.org/10.1001/archpsyc.61.11.1126.

13. Ehsan Pishva et al., "Epigenetic Genes and Emotional Reactivity to Daily Life Events: A Multi-Step Gene-Environment Interaction Study," edited by Yong-hui Dang, *PLOS ONE* 9, no. 6 (June 26, 2014): e100935, figure 1, 6, https://doi.org/10.1371/journal.pone.0100935.

GENE ANALYSIS FOR SKIN AND HEALTH

●●●●

DERMATOGENOMI X ®

BY Dr·Sharad™

BIOHACKING YOUR GENES

---

74 GENES TESTED

COMPREHENSIVE REPORT

HEALTH & WELLNESS

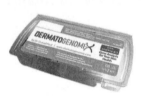

Understand your
genes and improve
your health and
well-being

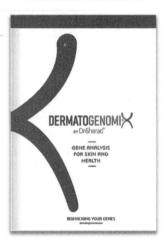

- Your personalized gene-test report will have diet and lifestyle recommendations

- The 74 genes that we test for are chosen specifically to help understand your physiology for health and wellness

- Knowledge about the skin-brain axis helps you understand your individual risk for many diseaes

- The Dermatogenomix® gene test is unique because it is not focused on any specific disease but in optimizing your wellness

Order now at:
WWW.BIOHACKINGYOURGENES.COM